A Sociology of
Hikikomori

A Sociology of Hikikomori

Experiences of Isolation, Family-Dependency, and Social Policy in Contemporary Japan

Teppei Sekimizu

LEXINGTON BOOKS
Lanham • Boulder • New York • London

Published by Lexington Books
An imprint of The Rowman & Littlefield Publishing Group, Inc.
4501 Forbes Boulevard, Suite 200, Lanham, Maryland 20706
www.rowman.com

86-90 Paul Street, London, EC2A 4NE

Originally published in 2016 as *'Hikikomori' Keiken no Shakaigaku* in Japanese

British Library Cataloguing in Publication Information Available

Library of Congress Cataloging-in-Publication Data

Names: Sekimizu, Teppei, author.
Title: A sociology of hikikomori : experiences of isolation, family-dependency, and social policy in contemporary Japan / Teppei Sekimizu.
Description: Lanham : Lexington Books, [2022] | Includes bibliographical references. | Summary: "Hikikomori is considered an increasingly prevalent form of social isolation in Japan. This book explores personal hikikomori experiences and explains how post-war Japanese social policy, which depends on corporations and families, has created several generations of isolated, family-dependent individuals in contemporary Japan"—Provided by publisher.
Identifiers: LCCN 2022023497 (print) | LCCN 2022023498 (ebook) | ISBN 9781666900941 (cloth) | ISBN 9781666900965 (paperback) | ISBN 9781666900958 (ebook)
Subjects: LCSH: Hikikomori. | Social isolation—Japan. | Social distance—Japan. | Japan—Social policy. | Japan—Social conditions—1945-
Classification: LCC HN723.5 .S345 2022 (print) | LCC HN723.5 (ebook) | DDC 302.5/450952—dc23/eng/20220519
LC record available at https://lccn.loc.gov/2022023497
LC ebook record available at https://lccn.loc.gov/2022023498

Contents

Acknowledgments

I would like to express my sincere gratitude to the Faculty of Social Welfare at Rissho University, which offered me the valuable opportunity of a one-year sabbatical from April 2021 to March 2022. I could devote all my time to my research and finish writing this book thanks to this.

Dr. Jochen Dreher, the executive director of the Social Science Archive Konstanz at the University of Konstanz, accepted me as a visiting scholar during my sabbatical and provided me with a comfortable laboratory and a great environment where I could concentrate on my research. He not only gave me advice on my research but also helped me with daily problems during my stay in Germany. I really appreciate his generous support.

I would also like to thank Dr. Anush Yeghiazaryan at the Social Science Archive Konstanz for her constant supportive attitude. I received a lot of intellectual stimulation during our conversations over coffee.

Dr. Jan Straßheim read my proposal for Lexington Books and gave me insightful comments. Thanks to him, I was able to brush up my proposal.

My gratitude also goes to Dan Alderson, who read the first draft of this book, checked my English, and gave me very warm comments to encourage me to complete it.

Timothy Eshing read the whole manuscript very carefully, making countless effective suggestions. His dedication really helped improve the final product. I also appreciate Professor Michael Barber of Saint Louis University for his warm support in introducing me to Timothy.

In Japan, Sachiko Horiguchi, professor at Temple University, Japan Campus, and Kiwako Endo, assistant professor at Kinjo Gakuin University, co-researchers of our ongoing international comparative study of hikikomori issue, provided invaluable support for my book project.

I'm grateful to Mr. Manabu Koyanagi, president of Japanese publisher, Sayu-sha, for publishing the Japanese version of this book on hikikomori in 2016 and kindly agreeing to publish this book as an English edition of the Japanese original.

Hisashi Nasu, professor emeritus of Waseda University, guided me as a mentor in my graduate years, connected me with the University of Konstanz, and led me to this publication. I could not have pursued my career as a sociologist without his generosity and patience.

Finally, I would also like to convey my gratitude to the many people who have experienced hikikomori and have generously spared their time to participate in my interview research, and the many people who have taught me various things during my fieldwork. I hope that this book will lead to a better understanding of their hikikomori experiences and their social contexts.

This work was supported by JSPS KAKENHI Grant Numbers 18K12949, 20K02194, 21K02004.

Glossary of Japanese Terms

80 50 [Hachimaru-Gōmaru] Mondai, the eighty-fifty problem

The problem in which parents in their 80s have to take care of their adult hikikomori children in their 50s.

Futōkō, School non-attendance

The condition in which elementary school children and junior and senior high-school students do not or cannot go to school; before the 1970s, the terms "truancy" (*Taigaku*) and "school phobia" (*Gakkō Kyōfu Shō*) were used to refer to this condition, but the term "school refusal" (*Tōkōkyohi*) became popular around the 1970s, and the term "school non-attendance" (*Futōkō*) has become more common since the 1990s.

Freeter

This Japanese English word was coined in the 1980s from "free" and "arbeiter" (viz., "worker" in German). It signifies a part-time, low-wage, precarious worker.

KHJ, KHJ National Federation of Families with Hikikomori

"KHJ National Federation of Families with Hikikomori" (*KHJ Zenkoku Hikikomori Kazoku-kai Rengōkai*). KHJ is an abbreviation for "Family [*Kazoku*], Hikikomori, Japan." This was originally established in 1999 as an association for parents with hikikomori children. It has 57 members as of 2021.

MHLW, Ministry of Health, Labour, and Welfare

The Ministry of Health, Labour and Welfare (MHLW) was established in 2001 by merging the Ministry of Health and Welfare (MHW) and the Ministry of Labour.

NEET, "Not in Education, Employment, or Training"

The concept of "NEET" was imported from the United Kingdom. The Japanese NEET is a modified version of the original NEET concept used in British youth policy since the 1990s. NEET in the United Kingdom was a concept to illuminate youths' "social exclusion," which included unemployment. However, the "Japanese NEET" concept described by Reiko Kosugi was to irradiate not "socially-excluded youth" but rather "those who are not participating in social activities and therefore may become a future cost to society and are not sufficiently activated by current employment support measures" (Kosugi 2004, 6).

Shūshoku Katsudō, a Japanese style of job-hunting

One of the characteristics of *Shūshoku Katsudō* in Japan is that companies and government offices hire those who are about to graduate from high school, vocational school, or university as *Sei-shain* (full-time employees) only once a year. In the *Shūshoku Katsudō* process for college students, they need to find a job between the end of their junior year and the end of their senior year, according to the hiring schedule of the company. If they receive an offer from a company, they will join the company soon after graduation in March.

Preface

Emergence of Hikikomori

The word "hikikomori" was included in the third edition of the *Oxford English Dictionary* (*OED*) in 2010. It defines a hikikomori as follows: hikikomori is "(in Japan) the extreme avoidance of social contact, especially by adolescent males," or "a person who avoids social contact."

It was actually in the late 1980s, more than 20 years before the *OED* included the word, that Japanese society began to pay attention to this phenomenon and began to use that term. When the issue of hikikomori first became known, the typical image of a hikikomori was that of a male who had been out of school, living with his parents into his 20s or 30s.

Initially, psychological counselors and psychiatrists discussed hikikomori, but in 2001, two books by hikikomori individuals were published: *Hikikomori Calendar* by Minoru Katsuyam in February and *From Me, Who Was a "Hikikomori"* by Kazuki Ueyama in December. The authors are both male, and they also fit into the typical image of hikikomori in the early 2000s.

Kazuki Ueyama was born in Kobe city in 1968. He was a sensitive child, good to his mother, and felt that he had to be an honor student in order to make a place for himself in the class. However, when he was around 14 years old, in the autumn of second year of junior high school, he was trying his best to study for the entrance exam for a better high school, but something strange happened. His head felt heavy as if it were made of lead, and he could not concentrate on his studies at all. From the summer break of his final year of junior high school, he was unable to go to school at all. Although he managed to enroll in high school, he could not bring himself to go. The feeling that he was "outside the gear device of the world" would not go away, and he dropped out during his second year of high school. After that, he tried going to college and finding a job, but no matter what he did, he could not "join society," and continued to live with his mother (Ueyama 2001).

Minoru Katsuyama was born in Yokohama city in 1971. Since he was a small child, he conformed to his mother's expectations, who expected him to be "perfect." He attended the high school his mother wanted. However, in high school, he felt that he could no longer continue to meet his mother's expectations and eventually refused to go to school, dropping out in his final year. After that, he failed his college entrance exams three times. At the age of 26, he feared he was going crazy and went to see a psychiatrist. After that, he stayed with his parents while he communicated on the Internet with people in similar situations (Katsuyama 2001).

Their experiences will be discussed in detail in the first chapter of this book, but what they experienced in common is deep disappointment and feelings of self-denial, as well as severe conflict with their parents, who expected them to go to school and work while financially supporting them. They blame themselves and are blamed by those around them.

Twenty years have passed since then. The Cabinet Office published a report in 2016 that showed the incidence of hikikomori cases among 15–39-year-olds is at 1.57% and the estimated number of hikikomori cases is 541,000 (Cabinet Office 2016).

From around 2010, the middle-aged and older hikikomori became a social topic, and from the latter half of 2010, people have been paying more attention to prolonged hikikomori cases. Furthermore, the hikikomori issue became connected with the "80 50 [*Hachimaru-Gōmaru*] problem," in which parents in their 80s have to take care of their adult hikikomori children in their 50s. Female hikikomori cases also gained attention in mass media.

In 2019, the Cabinet Office published a new hikikomori survey report which targeted the middle and older age group from 40 to 64 years old. It showed the incidence of hikikomori in the age group of 40–64-year-olds is 1.45% and the estimated number is 613,000 (Cabinet Office 2019a). The mass media reported that the number of hikikomori cases between the ages of 15 and 64 is estimated to be more than 1 million, along with the results of the 2016 survey report (Asahi Shinbun, evening edition, March 29, 2019).

Although the focus of society's attention changes from time to time, the attention paid to hikikomori has not yet waned in Japan; the mass media regularly mention the issue, and people continue to talk about it with interest. This issue has also attracted international attention, and, as mentioned previously, in 2010 the revised edition of the *Oxford English Dictionary* included the word "hikikomori."

OVERVIEW OF MY FIELD RESEARCH
ON HIKIKOMORI

I began to research the hikikomori issue in the mid-2000s. My interest was sparked by a book published by Ueyama in 2001. His philosophical stance in trying to verbalize how he felt the world's injustice toward him overlapped with the difficulty I experienced in my own life in Japanese society. I went on to study sociology in graduate school and began research on the hikikomori experience and its social backgrounds.

In the mid-2000s, I started participating in a group of hikikomori subjects, parents with hikikomori children, support professionals and researchers, which was held in the Tokyo metropolitan area. It had been held since the early 2000, and in the mid-2000s, there were about 20 participants each time. At the beginning of each meeting, everyone did a brief self-introduction, and then talked about a specific theme, though sometimes they had free talk. It seemed to me that most of the hikikomori people wanted to share their sufferings and that most parents attended the meeting because they wanted to learn what their hikikomori children were thinking and feeling, and what they could do about it.

I've now been involved in the group for more than 15 years, and I have interviewed hikikomori people I met at the meeting. I asked them to introduce me to other hikikomori people, and thus far, I have interviewed more than 20 hikikomori people. I have also interviewed parents who lived with hikikomori children in the Tokyo metropolitan area.

While referring to the experiences of hikikomori people and parents of hikikomori children I met throughout this book, I will focus on the narratives of six hikikomori people in table 0.1.

DEFINITION OF TERMS: HIKIKOMORI
SUBJECTS, HIKIKOMORI EXPERIENCE,
AND HIKIKOMORI PROBLEMS

I began my hikikomori research with an interest in the subjective experience of the hikikomori state, but when I first started participating in support group meetings, I was puzzled by the diversity of hikikomori people. The stories they told at the meeting ranged from the experience of bullying at school, the pain of working, the feelings of self-denial, current and future financial insecurities, resentment toward parents, and the lack of a place to stay. Not a few of them had diagnoses of mental disorders, for example, depression, developmental disorder, adjustment disorder, and borderline personality disorder. Despite their adoption of the "hikikomori" label, which

Table 0.1   List of Interviewees

Name	Year of Birth	Profile	Interview Date
Mr. A	Early 1980s	He could not go job-hunting when he graduated university. Since then, he had stayed at home for one year.	July 15, 2015
Mr. B	Early 1970s	He was bullied in elementary school and high school. After he graduated university, he worked as part-timer, then he withdrew for two years.	February 27, 2012 March 5, 2012
Mr. C	Late 1970s	He did not go to school from the elementary level onward and lived mainly at home with his parents while he saw psychotherapists and psychiatrists.	February 11, 2012 April 15, 2012
Ms. D	Late 1960s	She dropped out of high school and worked as part-timer for several years. After that, she withdrew for two years.	March 17, 2012
Mr. E	Early 1980s	He stopped going to school when he was in the first year of junior high. He worked as part-timer, but he also had mental problems and stayed home for several short periods.	April 17, 2010
Mr. F	Late 1960s	He was unable to attend high school and repeated the first year four times. After graduating university, he worked as a high-school teacher for a year, and then withdrew for seven years.	November 16, 2008 (Field notes)
Minoru Katsuyama	1971	After he dropped out of high school and tried to enroll university, he tried to work as part-timer, but found he could not. He lived at home with his parents for many years while receiving a disability pension.	June 30, 2010 June 30, 2011 August 23, 2011

means a person who stays in a room or house or his/her state, the percentage of individuals who leave home was also larger than I'd expected. Some hikikomori people said they basically lived their lives without leaving their homes, while others could go out to meet others or worked as part-timers.

This book considers people who define themselves as hikikomori and/or define their past or present experience as hikikomori. It does not adopt objective definitions (such as those proposed by psychiatrists) but instead accepts the self-definition of such people. The most crucial reason for this approach is that the idea of hikikomori is originally not an item of scientific knowledge, which scientists determine, but rather an item of everyday knowledge whose meaning develops through usage in everyday contexts. The state of hikikomori experienced by the hikikomori subjects in this book does not necessarily fit the definition proposed by psychiatrists. The self-defined hikikomori in everyday knowledge is not aligned with the definitions by experts, but does interact with them (see chapter 2).

This book does not make a clear distinction between those who have experienced hikikomori state in the past and those who are currently in a hikikomori state. Both are referred to as hikikomori subjects in this book. According to subjective definitions of hikikomori, it is often difficult to determine exactly when a state of hikikomori begins and ends. Hikikomori people are also uncertain if or when they would fall into a state of hikikomori again. Thus, it is not easy to distinguish past from a present hikikomori state. In everyday Japanese language, the term "individuals in a hikikomori state [*hikikomori tōjisha*]" also often refers to both those who have experienced hikikomori state in the past and those who are currently experiencing a state of hikikomori. This ambiguity of terminology sometimes leads to debates about who is a legitimate hikikomori subject and what is a legitimate state of hikikomori—even among hikikomori subjects.[1]

In terms of parents with hikikomori children, listening to their stories, I often felt that the problems that they faced were different from the existential problem experienced by hikikomori subjects. Families had a variety of concerns, such as how to communicate with hikikomori children, their inability to continue working, and the uncertain economic future of their households. In addition, mass media and policy makers predominantly discuss the problems of hikikomori from the perspective of the family and Japanese society, emphasizing the burden on the public assistance system or how society can provide financial and/or employment support for hikikomori cases and families with hikikomori children, but they rarely focus on hikikomori subjects' first-personal experiences and the existential problems they face.

To explore the hikikomori phenomenon, this book clearly distinguishes the "hikikomori experience" as the first-personal experience of a hikikomori state by hikikomori subjects from the "hikikomori problem" as a social issue for society and families with hikikomori children, and it approaches both topics from separate angles. When it refers to both aspects of the hikikomori experience and the hikikomori problem, it uses the term "hikikomori phenomenon."

Related to the aforementioned text, there is often a discrepancy between the self-definition of hikikomori used by hikikomori subjects and the definition of hikikomori used by others. Sometimes families complain that their hikikomori children do not recognize that they are in a hikikomori state. This discrepancy lies between subjective (the first personal) and objective (the third personal) usages of the term "hikikomori."

Therefore, this book uses "hikikomori subjects/people/individuals" when it is in accordance with self-identification of people in such a state (i.e., from the subjective perspective) and use "hikikomori cases/children" when others define a person as hikikomori from outside a state of hikikomori (i.e., the objective perspective in that sense). If neither the subjective nor the objective usage is specified, it uses "withdrawn people," "people in withdrawal," or simply "a hikikomori."

OBJECTS AND METHODS OF ANALYSIS

As explained earlier, the hikikomori phenomenon has at least two essentially different aspects: the first-personal hikikomori experience of the hikikomori subjects and the third-personal hikikomori problem for the family or society (e.g., policy makers and mass media).

Thus, we can consider three units to which the hikikomori phenomenon appears differently: hikikomori subjects, the family, and society. We can identify hikikomori phenomena for each unit. Of course, it is impossible to isolate, for example, hikikomori people's experience purely from that of the family or society, as they intrinsically relate to one another, but it is possible to isolate those aspects as the focus of analysis.

As table 0.2 displays, each chapter in this book analyzes a different aspect of the overall hikikomori phenomenon with a different theoretical framework.

Chapter 1 deals with the first-personal hikikomori experience for hikikomori people. A hikikomori subject, Kazuki Ueyama, says that hikikomori is a question. This chapter will decipher what it means for the hikikomori experience to be a kind of question.

Chapter 2 also deals with the hikikomori experience but focuses on the term "hikikomori" and its usage to define oneself: the process of self-categorization as a hikikomori subject and the process of becoming a hikikomori subject is explored via Ian Hacking's concept of "human kinds."

Chapter 3 identifies what the hikikomori problem is for families based on statistical data and examines the social structural contexts in which the

Table 0.2   List of Subjects and Methods in Each Chapter

	Subject of Analysis	*Method of Analysis*
Chapter 1	Hikikomori Experience	Phenomenological approach
Chapter 2	Hikikomori Experience	Sociology of knowledge approach
Chapter 3	Hikikomori Problems for Family	Welfare regime theory
Chapter 4	Hikikomori Problems for Society	Discourse analysis
Chapter 5	Hikikomori Experience	Interaction theory
Chapter 6	Hikikomori Experience	Narrative theory

third-personal hikikomori problem for family arises and is sustained. This chapter also focuses on the relationship between families with hikikomori children and society.

Chapter 4 focuses on the hikikomori problem for society (e.g., policy makers, mass media, and psychiatrists). It summarizes what has been said about the hikikomori problem, focusing on government policy texts, mass media reports, and psychiatrists' discourses from the 1980s to 2020.

Chapter 5 again treats the first-personal hikikomori experience, with particular attention paid to their participation in social interactions. It explores what creates difficulties of participation, clarified by examining Erik H. Erikson's theory of self-identity and Erving Goffman's theory of the situational self. It also discusses how to best provide support for hikikomori people.

Chapter 6 discusses hikikomori subjects themselves. The focal points are on the narrative wreckage in their hikikomori experience and the retelling process of their life stories. It also considers the difference between Anthony Giddens' concepts of discursive and practical consciousness.

Each chapter can be read independently, but reading through all chapters will help readers understand the different aspects of the hikikomori phenomenon (the hikikomori experience and hikikomori as a social problem) and the social structural backgrounds of this phenomenon. The hikikomori experience, which is largely defined by the unique context of Japanese society, is an experience of isolation and a search for a relationship with society and with oneself. The hikikomori problem for family and society also reflects the uniqueness of Japanese society. Thus, we will gain a better understanding of the characteristics of Japanese society through exploration of the hikikomori phenomenon. However, this book will also clarify a universal aspect of social isolation in the experience of hikikomori and universal social structural conditions of the hikikomori problem that hold true across societies.

NOTE

1. This discussion is called the "false hikikomori controversy" (*Nise-Hiki Ronsō*) (Nico Nico Pedia 2022). Ishikawa (2007, 128) also mentions this term.

Chapter 1

The Hikikomori Experience and Ambivalence

This chapter examines the hikikomori experience, focusing on the key questions which hikikomori subjects ask and are asked. Kazuki Ueyama, a hikikomori subject, states as follows: "Hikikomori is, first and foremost, a question. It is a very easy answer to say 'you have to work' or 'you have to go to school.' Instead of unconditionally imposing such 'answers,' please share the questions. Hikikomori is first and foremost a 'question' for the hikikomori subjects themselves. I ask their families to share their 'question'" (Ueyama 2001, 107).

What is the "question" that Ueyama refers to? This chapter will clarify what questions are asked by the hikikomori experience. The argument proceeds as follows. The next section will confirm the meaning of the question by examining Ueyama's hikikomori experience as written in his book *From Me Who Was "Hikikomori"* (Ueyama 2001). Then, the following three sections take up the narratives of five hikikomori subjects and analyze how they experience the questions based on their interview data. Finally, the question in the hikikomori experience will be examined theoretically through H. Arendt's perspective on "appearance."

QUESTIONS AND AMBIVALENCE IN THE HIKIKOMORI EXPERIENCE

Questions in the Hikikomori Experience of Kazuki Ueyama

Although there is no clear definition of question in his book, the following statements give us an important clue to understand what he means:

> I think that contemporary society demands *responding* in a very hasty manner.
> . . . It seems in the same context to adhere to the *response*: "We must work

1

anyhow." They never take the *question* seriously, and they cannot envision any other way of living than earning a living by immediately responding to *given questions* in front of them. . . . *Given questions*—yes, I feel this is fundamental. We are forced to respond to *given questions*, not *self-addressed questions.* (Ueyama 2001, 185)

Here Ueyama contrasts "given questions" with "self-addressed questions." The former are irresistible questions which are asked by others. They are not genuine questions, but rhetorical ones. They have predetermined answers: "Why don't you work? (You have to work)," "What are you going to do? (You have to do something)." Those questions are immediately directed at hikikomori subjects who have deviated from the expected life course.

On the other hand, self-addressed questions do not have ready-made answers like the given questions of others. As Ueyama explains, the hikikomori condition itself is an enigma for hikikomori subjects because it is not their intentional choice. Hikikomori people find themselves in the hikikomori condition against their will. And then they confront their own questions: "Why am I in this situation?" or "What can or should I do from here?" These are questions which the hikikomori subjects have to ask themselves in their hikikomori state.

These self-addressed questions involve a unique ambivalence. Ueyama describes "a typical ambivalence of hikikomori subjects" as follows:

I am suffering from a tremendous sense of "injustice" regarding my past and my surroundings—the people I have encountered, especially my family. When I go to a third person for advice, such as psychiatrists, all they say is, "Don't dwell on the past," "It's your own fault," or "You must change your mind," but they never say anything sympathetic about my frustration   On the one hand, "I know I am out of step with the standard of this society and saying crazy things," but on the other hand, "there must be something in the injustice I feel." (Ueyama 2001, 146)

Ueyama expresses his contradictory feelings, like both "I am wrong" and "I am not wrong." The former feeling, "I am wrong," is rooted in his disposition to live up to the expectations of others. His hikikomori state is totally deviant from others' expectations, and he has to deny himself as maladjusted. On the other hand, the latter feeling, "I am not wrong," derives from his attitude in response to others' expectations and a desire to respect his own nature. These are ambivalent feelings because what is required to respect his own nature contradicts what is required to meet the expectations of others.

Ueyama understands this ambivalence as balancing the response to others' requirements with the adjustment to his own mind. He argues that such balance is what is lost in the hikikomori experience. Hikikomori individuals are imbalanced: they cannot moderate between others' reality and their own (Ueyama 2001, 190).

Thus, what Ueyama means by confronting the self-addressed questions is not being dominated by others' expectations, but rather to respect their own nature and confront this ambivalence and seek for balancing between them. Yasuhiko Maruyama, an experienced counselor who experienced the hikikomori condition himself, formulates the ambivalence in the hikikomori experience clearly and formulates it as a process of integrating the "wishing" (*Negai*) to meet the expectations of others, and the "longing" (*Omoi*) to live without bending one's own true feelings (Maruyama 2014).

Thus, the questions in the hikikomori experience can be classified as in table 1.1. The largest category is "imposed questions." This includes every type of question hikikomori subjects experience and is divided into two subcategories: given questions and self-addressed questions. The former literally consists of the questions that others—for example, parents, teachers, psychiatrists—ask hikikomori subjects. The latter consists of the questions to which they have to find their own answers, which contain ambivalence between responding to others' expectations and respecting their own nature.

However, Ueyama also describes self-addressed questions as follows: "Being 'hikikomori' may begin as an opportunity to take a short distance from the violent and merciless *interrogations* and to reexamine *self-addressed questions* (and then realize that the *questions* indeed have no place in society, and one gets more and more stuck . . .)" (Ueyama 2001, 186). Confronting self-addressed questions requires stepping back from the questions of others, yet hikikomori people realize that self-addressed questions "have no place in society." Why is this so?

Despair in Communication

Regarding the ambivalence of self-addressed questions, the disposition to respond to others' expectations is easily understood by the people around hikikomori subjects. On the other hand, it is difficult for people who have never experienced the hikikomori state to respect and comprehend their own nature and the feeling of injustice of hikikomori subjects because hikikomori is nothing more than something to be denied for those people.

Table 1.1   Multiple Questions in the Hikikomori Experience

	Imposed Questions	
	Self-Addressed Questions	
Given Questions (Questions of Others)	Responding to expectations from others	Respecting one's own nature

When other people do not understand the ambivalence between responding to others' expectations and respecting their own nature, hikikomori people become thoroughly isolated. He describes this isolation as follows: "There is no one around me who understands the structure of my ponderous dilemma and ambivalence. However, these *people who don't understand me* collude to form a *society* and work to create their *living*, and . . . there is nothing I can do" (Ueyama 2001, 147).

This misrecognition of the ambivalence also leads to "despair in communication." Ueyama writes: "In short, they have a radical despair in communication," and "There is no human voice to be heard from anywhere" (Ueyama 2001, 141). He also described a significant feeling he had, that his voice—and his voice alone—was being excluded (Ueyama 2001, 142). There is no one who understands the ambivalence in the self-addressed questions, and one is surrounded by the questions of others.

This isolation and despair in communication hinder the hikikomori subjects' (1) recognition and acceptance of their own nature, and (2) balancing of respect for their own nature with responding to the expectations of others. However, these two explorations seem to be essential parts of self-addressed questions. In the situation where they tend to be dominated by the questions of others, how do they regard these self-addressed questions and what are they confronting in the questions?

FIVE CASES OF THE HIKIKOMORI EXPERIENCE

The Case of Mr. A

This section clarifies how hikikomori people experience the self-addressed questions connected with the ambivalence by examining the experiences of five hikikomori subjects based mainly on interview data. Five of them are Mr. A, Mr. B, Mr. C, Ms. D, and Minoru Katsuyama.

The first case, Mr. A, was born in the early 1980s. During a job-hunting period of his senior year at university, he lost his motivation and stayed home for about a year, mostly lying in bed, and subsequently fell into a hikikomori condition for about six years.

> During the six years of withdrawal, I spent about 15 hours a day watching internet streaming and playing games. The reason why I was in such a state was because I was not good at finding a job. I did a little job-hunting, but I found it wasn't for me. I got stuck in a deadlock and went to bed for about a year. Retrospectively thinking about it, I might have been depressed. I must have enjoyed my college years quite a bit. I did job-hunting [*Shūshoku Katsudō*] for a bit, but I found it tough for me and gave up on getting a job. Eventually, I started staying at home.

. . . It's difficult when you leave the normal path of graduating from university and getting a job. I think everyone [upon the normal path] is great.

He experienced conflict over his inability at *Shūshoku Katsudō*, or Japanese-style job-hunting. He says, "I must have enjoyed my college years quite a bit," but the job-hunting was difficult for him.

> I've had part-time jobs and temporary jobs [during university days]. But job-hunting was different. I still don't want to do that. I sometimes feel heavy to go to work, but I don't think I dislike working itself. That's still the case. I think I don't like job-hunting, maybe. . . . Even if I had done job-hunting and had started working, it would have been difficult. I don't think I'd be able to continue working if the working conditions are too severe. The appeal of being normal is huge, though.

He himself did not know why he was so unable to pursue job-hunting. In this respect, his hikikomori condition was also an "imposed question" for him. The imposed question, "Why can't I pursue job-hunting?" was initially overshadowed by the self-denying thought. He was also entranced with given questions from others which already had the answer: "I must do job-hunting and find a full-time job." He says, "While I was hikikomori, I had the feeling that not working meant I was not human."

However, Mr. A gradually recognized the ambivalence through reading books written by Minoru Katsuyama, a hikikomori person, and Mr. Pha, a *NEET*, who both tried to affirm a life without working and through online communications with other hikikomori subjects. These encounters were the earliest experiences by which he learned of approaches that did not deny his maladjustment. In Ueyama's words, "There must be something in the injustice I feel." Through them, he could feel that "this kind [of life] can be possible" and "I can manage my life somehow."

Although he had a very strong sense of self-denial that "not working meant I was not human," he came to reexamine the imposed question and started to explore his own nature and his own balancing of the requirements from others with being faithful to his own nature. This question has no ready-made answer. He is still questioning himself: Is there really no way of living if I cannot do job hunting to attain a full-time job?

The Case of Mr. B

Mr. B was born in the early 1970s. He experienced bullying in the upper grades of elementary school and was ignored by all of his classmates after the summer break of his first year of high school. He managed to graduate from high school and studied for one year for the college entrance exam, then he went on to college. Although he pursued job-hunting in the final year of university, he was unable to find a full-time job, and continued to work part-time after graduation. He worked as a part-timer for about a year, then he was fired. He experienced a similar situation twice in a row, and this experience made him unable to work. He said: "I was behaving normally, but people were giving me negative feedback. I thought I was dumb. I didn't know how to act anymore. I was just confused and didn't know what to do anymore. What I could do was only breathing. There was nothing I could do."

Mr. B referred to the reason why he suddenly became afraid of working as follows:

> I guess I felt like I was being denied. I couldn't take a rational point of view that the fact I couldn't get a job was just a fact of being job-less, but I felt like I was being denied my entire personality and existence. That was what I felt for a while. Anyway, I didn't know what was going on, in my 20s. I still don't understand it, but it used to be even more foggy. When I think about it now, I didn't understand myself, I didn't recognize myself, I was in a fog. My mind was sinking in a depressed feeling, or I just felt like I was frightened all the time.

Trapped in self-denial, questions from others besieged him: "Why can't I keep working normally?"

> Why can't I do things normally, am I crazy? But I didn't think I was sick, so I just wondered why. If I could figure it out, I would still have the courage to try again, but I didn't at that time, and I felt like I was doomed. When I was in college, or when I was a *Freeter* at first, I thought that I just happened to be not in the right place at the right time, and that there was a place for me. . . . I was sure that I had completely lost my energy by the time I was 25. I couldn't move anymore. I couldn't get a job or a part-time job. I didn't even want to meet people.

He did not know why he could not keep working. After losing his job, Mr. B spent two years in his mid-twenties hardly leaving his home. He answered the question "What did you think about during that time?" as follows:

> Actually, I didn't think. I didn't think about the future. It was just a resentment. Mostly resentment from elementary school, junior high school, and high school. "Because of him . . ." Ah, yes, passing the buck. "It's their fault, the ones who bullied me." I don't know why but I brought up the resentments for people who bullied me again. And then there was a cycle, like parents, teachers, then bosses. But parents and bosses not so often. [More] the ones who bullied me, I

guess. In elementary, junior high, high school, and in college, those with whom I experienced strained [relationships]. Also, those who I got into trouble within the workplace. Even with a co-worker: "He was such a jerk." I think that was the biggest part of that time.

As Ueyama pointed out, the despair in the present leads a hikikomori subject to cling to the past. Mr. B longingly ruminated on the past while he was surrounded by the given questions of others, which pressured him to think about the future.

He experienced a complex feeling regarding people who were in a similar condition with him. Although he was living mainly at home and in a hikikomori condition objectively, he did not think of himself a hikikomori.

> Although I watched some special TV programs on the hikikomori issue, I looked down on them, despised those people. I thought I was different from them. It was a strange phenomenon. In the beginning, it was on the evening news programs or NHK. . . . I think subconsciously I was looking for a place to stand or my position, but I couldn't reach that deeper level of consciousness and couldn't see myself in that situation. So, on the surface, I was looking down on them, and I was relying on my baseless confidence that "I'm not like them, I'm in this condition, but I'll come out of it, I'll be okay." I was very conscious of the thought that "I just happen to be like this now. I'm different from them."

He could not accept himself as a hikikomori, although he "subconsciously" wanted to position himself as a hikikomori person. He proceeded to talk about exploration of his nature as follows:

> But gradually, in my late 20s, I started to actively watch programs about hikikomori, and while superficially still thinking that I was different, I tried to get information. I can't really describe the change, though. It was a natural change. Since I was physically in my room and had no contact with society, my information from the outside was limited. I don't know what to call it. I guess you could call it self-acceptance. Although, I think I had differentiated myself from other hikikomori subjects somehow.

In the beginning, he kept denying his maladjustment and looked down on hikikomori subjects. This thought accords with the rhetorical questions from others, "Why don't you work? (You must work)," which surrounded him.

However, Mr. B becomes aware of an affirmative perspective of the maladjusted self by watching a TV documentary about hikikomori subjects. He says:

> The people who came to the place [in the documentary program] did not seem sick, so everyone was in harmony, and it was not like they were limping around. It seemed like they were taking a break and looking for the next step or stage. I thought, "Oh, such a place exists," and then I thought, "Let me look for one in Tokyo" and "I thought that if I could go to such a place, I would be able to be a little more natural even if I were not cured."

After a long period of denying his own inability to meet the demands of those around him, he began to recognize his own existence and his own questions concerning the balance between meeting the demands of others and respecting his own nature. He gradually identified himself as a hikikomori subject, and he joined a support group for hikikomori people. Since then, Mr. B has participated in several hikikomori support groups and is currently living at home while working part-time.

The Case of Mr. C

Mr. C was born in the late 1970s. He had difficulty in joining groups since kindergarten. He entered elementary school but stopped going to school around the summer break of his first year. He said, "I didn't want to be in the classroom, or rather, I couldn't be in the classroom."

> I really used up my engine or energy. I was afraid too much, my anxiety got too great, and I couldn't keep myself going. Because I had a strong anticipatory anxiety, I thought about the future, and I was worried about what would happen next. Unexpected things happened, and then I was not able to keep myself going.

Although Mr. C didn't actually attend elementary and junior high school, he graduated from them.[1] He then attended a correspondence high school, but his nervousness increased when he went out. When he got on a train to go to school, he repeatedly got off on the way because of strain and stomach problems. Currently, he is working part-time as a building cleaner, but he does not find it easy to do so.

> I do the utmost to work, and even though it's only two and a half hours of work in the evening, it takes up the whole day. I can't do anything else. After all, I am so nervous about going to work. I'm afraid whether I would be able to get on a train. . . . I'm also worried that if I couldn't go to work, I would be fired. The people around me don't understand me, and they don't understand how much to keep working means for me, how and why I feel so desperate and overwhelmed.

As people around him questioned why he would not go to school as people usually do, he could not accept that he was not able to comply with the expected way of life.

> Yes, after all, I had only a negative perspective during my hikikomori condition. I had to start from accepting myself as a school non-attendance [*Futōkō*]. . . . It is truly painful that I have to accept that. After all, I had to accept my incompetency. It's like, "I can do it, I can do anything, but why don't you understand me?" I want other people to understand that I can do it, but the truth is that I can't do it. So, after all, [I have to recognize] myself as being incompetent.

He did not acknowledge what he could do and what he could not do. Insisting "I can do it" was just trying to turn over the self-denial, and it was still premised on the denial of his incompetence. In order not to deny and to recognize what he is, he argues, he needs someone who listens to him without denying him or advising him: "When I have someone whom I can report to, speak to, someone who just listens to me, I gradually come to understand myself." He came to accept his inability to adapt to the expected life course of others. He says: "I came to accept that it is me who is incompetent, and that it is me who is always upset."

Mr. C's long period of self-denial was also a period in which he learned to recognize and accept his own nature. He gradually came to understand himself as a person who has a different style of adaptation to society, although, as he said, it was "truly painful that I have to accept that." He says: "The period of hikikomori was the time I realized that my adaptation to society was different from others and that I couldn't do the same things as everyone." His self-addressed question is "what is my own style of adaptation to society?" and it has no ready-made answer.

He worked on his self-addressed questions: who and what he is and how to balance the incompetent self with having social life. Currently, he still suffers from a lack of understanding from those around him about his nature, and he continues to struggle to find a way to balance his nature and his work.

The Case of Ms. D

Ms. D was born in the late 1960s. She did not appreciate the policy of the high school she entered, where, at the entrance ceremony, the school president declared the remaining days until the university entrance exam. Her classmates did not understand her discomfort, and her health gradually deteriorated. After transferring to a correspondence high school, she passed the University Entrance Qualification Examination and entered a university but dropped out again because she could not adjust to the university environment. After that, she continued to work part-time, feeling "the difficulty in life" (*ikidurasa*). In her mid-20s, she spent almost two years shut-in at home.

After her 20s, which she says were "just painful," she became aware of the term "hikikomori" through a series of articles in the *Asahi Shinbun*, a nationwide newspaper, and began to participate in a self-help group for hikikomori people. She describes that period as follows:

I realized that I really didn't like crowded trains through commuting [for one year] and I felt like I worked on accepting myself case by case as someone who can't live a normal life. It's like self-awareness. This [self-awareness] was [possible] because I encountered many people who understood me at the Y [a self-help group for hikikomori people]. Another reason was that in the counseling sessions with Dr. Z [a psychiatrist], he said, "The way you need to focus on is not that way, but this way." When I tried to go back to the main street, he said, "It's not that way. You should cherish the part of your life that your antenna has picked up, which you call 'the difficulty in life' [*ikidurasa*]." To be more specific, he kept saying in many episodes and stories for years, "You should cherish [the part of] yourself who thinks 'I don't want to ride on a crowded train, it's like livestock, and it's wrong as a living thing to be able to ride on such a crowded train.'" I realized that if I recognized that way, it would mean that I had to accept that I couldn't do what everyone else could do. I still hoped to go back to the original path, to be the same as everyone else. I thought that I could do that, that it could happen to me. But I was giving up on that. Dr. Z, he called it minority, kept telling me that "the way you should walk on is to make the most of your minority being," because I kept wanting to go back to this [majority] way.

At the hikikomori support group, Ms. D met people who understood her "difficulty in life," and was encouraged by a psychiatrist who repeatedly advised her not to deny her inability to adapt to the mainstream life course, but rather to cherish who and what she is.

Through these relations, she came to accept her "minority" (unconventional) self as what she is, as her own nature.[2] Although she remained ambivalent and retained a desire to go back to the "main street" of the majority path, Ms. D gradually came to accept her unconventional path as a "minority" through her 20s and 30s. Currently in her 40s, she lives with her husband, who has also experienced the hikikomori state and since the 2010s, she has been working as an activist to change society, which does not accept diverse unconventional ways of living.

The Case of Minoru Katsuyama

Minoru Katsuyama published a book in 2001, the same year as Kazuki Ueyama, about his experience as a hikikomori subject. However, compared to Ueyama, he asserts "I am not wrong" more strongly.

Katsuyama was raised by a father who was a "supremacist of the normal" (Katsuyama 2001, 49) and a mother who not only "demanded good scores in exams" but also "demanded perfection as a human being." She violated him mentally and physically if he did not meet her perfectionist expectations. He was a "filial son who completely fulfilled his parents' wishes" until he dropped out of high school (Katsuyama 2001, 20–23).

Growing up in such a family environment, Katsuyama "couldn't imagine anything other than [a life course] from a good school to a good company," and he "made desperate efforts to survive" (Katsuyama 2001, 6). He went to a progressive high school as his mother hoped. However, as soon as he entered the school, he "burned out completely," found it difficult to get up in the morning, and could not understand lectures in high school. His mother's "fussing" to "get him back on the elite course" was in vain, and in the end he had to drop out in his third year of high school because his attendance was not sufficient (Katsuyama 2001, 22–25).

From then on, Katsuyama entered a long period of hikikomori state. He bought a recruitment magazine of part-time jobs "under the illusion that I would return to society," and, six months later, he "mustered up the courage" to apply for a part-time job as a mailman. However, he quit the job after only two weeks. He describes his thoughts immediately after that event as follows: "After that, my hikikomori got worse. Loss of self-confidence. I'm afraid of people. I'm plagued every day by an obsession that I must work. When I sleep, I have nightmares about school. I blame myself" (Katsuyama 2001, 155).

Katsuyama kept blaming himself for dropping out for many years. However, he came to accept his own nature and adopt an "I am not wrong" stance. He wrote:

> Stay indoors. I think this is the best way to fight. Destroy the respectability [*Sekentei*], make a blank on my resume, and say goodbye to a good company. I need time to take back my life as my own, which I've lived as others told me. I'm so exhausted. I'll sleep for hours. By doing nothing, I'll crush the selfish expectations and wishes from idiots. I need a reset. It's okay to be unplugged. Empty myself out and start again from scratch. Don't be stingy. Throw away all the knowledge I've gained through memory training and start from zero. Let me throw away all my qualifications and educational background. Let me become a person with nothing. I feel anxious about being no one. It frightens me. In the end, I have to realize that everything of me is not mine. I have nothing. I want

to go back to the rail track. But that's a shame. I want to be what no one forces
me to be. That is the only way for me to truly live my life. My soul is hurting
so much. I just want to be myself without phoniness. However, how many more
decades can I survive? (Katsuyama 2001, 16–17)

Although Katsuyama's expressions show his anxiety, such as "I want to
go back to the [majority] rail track" or "how many more decades can I
survive?" he outstandingly tries to affirm his maladjusted self as who and
what he is. Katsuyama also says that hikikomori people are "fighting society
in the hardest way" (Katsuyama 2001, 163). It is a fight against parents who
demand them to "keep up their respectability" and a fight against "society"
that demands only "people who are willing to endure" (Katsuyama 2001,
13–17, 160–163).

Katsuyama's will to affirm himself is firm and clear because he gave up
his endurance to conform to the expectations of others after long years of
his mother's incessant harsh demands. He realized that "I can't endure it
anymore" from the bottom of his heart. He wrote: "This society imposes on
me a disgusting level of endurance and insists that it is normal. But I came to
know clearly that I couldn't endure it. I can't endure it anymore" (Katsuyama
2001, 150).

He deeply renounced responding to the demands of others who refuse to
recognize his own nature, and this stance formed his new starting point. He
wrote: "We live in an age where we can't get anything out of doing what
society assumes is good. It's all a lie that if we could get this certification, if
we could graduate from this school, and if we could join this company [all
will be well]. Then, what should we do? We live in an age where there is no
answer to this question" (Katsuyama 2001, 159). Katsuyama began "to take
back [his] life as [his] own" by radically examining the questions of others
and attempted to explore his self-addressed questions with no ready-made
answers, by moving in the direction of valuing the affirmation of his own
nature.

DISCUSSION OF AMBIVALENCE
FROM ARENDT'S PERSPECTIVE

This chapter has examined six hikikomori subjects: Ueyama, Mr. A, Mr.
B, Mr. C, Ms. D, and Katsuyama. All of them experienced a strong sense
of self-denial because of maladjustment to the life course expected by
others. However, they gradually came to recognize their own self-addressed
questions: recognizing their own nature and the balance between meeting the
expectations of others and accepting who and what they are. They differ as

to how much they emphasize each of these two aspects. Among them, Ms. D and Katsuyama put stronger emphasis on the latter aspect of this ambivalence (accepting who and what they are), whereas the others put more emphasis on the former aspect (meeting the expectations of others).

This section will discuss the process by which hikikomori subjects become aware of the ambivalence of their own questions on a more theoretical level by way of Hannah Arendt's phenomenological concept of "appearances." Arendt argues that the human reality is supported by others who accept one's experience. She expresses this in the following way: "The presence of others who see what we see and hear what we hear assures us of the reality of the world and ourselves" (Arendt [1958] 1998: 50).[3] Others' objective perspective assures us of the common reality of our world.

To transpose private experience into public, storytelling and talking about the private experiences are essential. As Schutz and Luckmann argued, language is a "socially objectivated system of meaning" (Schutz and Luckmann 1973, 234). Thus, the verbalization of an experience assures us that the experience can be a common reality, seen and heard by others.[4]

When we cannot find the words to talk about an experience, or when others do not see or hear our storytelling, the appearance of an experience as a common reality becomes difficult. In those situations, thoughts, feelings, and even perceptions will drift and remain "an uncertain, shadowy kind of existence" (Arendt [1958] 1998, 50).[5] Those thoughts, feelings, and perceptions that are obvious to others tend to acquire reality, while those which others neither see nor hear and thus do not appear to others remain more uncertain and shadowy experiences.

The nature of hikikomori subjects is not obvious even to themselves from the beginning. Rather, as they drop out of others' expected life course, they are seen as maladjusted, and it becomes difficult for them to see their existence in a different way. However, as this chapter has discussed, the hikikomori subjects gradually confirm their own nature through various encounters—such as books, Internet communication, TV programs, and communication with psychiatrists.

Through this self-recognition process, they face the question of how to balance responding to the demands of others with respecting their own nature. It is also difficult for hikikomori subjects to recognize their ambivalence apparently because, among the myriad experiences of hikikomori subjects, only thoughts of self-denial and feelings of maladjustment are easily seen and heard by others, and the self-affirmative aspects of their experience are too rarely seen and heard, and thus deprived of appearance.

Hikikomori subjects are looking for others who can recognize their own nature as it is and bear witness to their ambivalence. As quoted at the beginning of this chapter, Ueyama said, "Instead of unconditionally imposing such 'answers,' please share the questions." Mr. C also said, "When I have someone whom I can report to, speak to, someone who just listens to me, I gradually come to understand myself." All hikikomori subjects discussed in this chapter have talked about their encounters with those witnesses who share their ambivalent experience. These others who make appearance possible are not limited to those in face-to-face interactions but include various relationships with media representations.

The hikikomori experience is a dynamic process of coming to know the nature of oneself, of accepting who and what one is, and determining how to balance who and what one is with the expectations from others. Just as Mr. C became aware that his approach of adapting to society is different from others' and began to explore his own style of social participation, the hikikomori experience as a set of self-addressed questions involves a process of trial and error without any ready-made answers.

CONCLUSION

This chapter has clarified the questions that define the hikikomori experience. Our examinations of the hikikomori cases show that their self-addressed questions involve the process of self-recognition and ambivalence about the hikikomori self. It is also not a straightforward process for them to recognize and articulate their own nature and their ambivalence. This process is undertaken not only through face-to-face interactions but also through online communications and reading books.

Although all of us—not only hikikomori subjects—experience this ambivalence between meeting the expectations of others and being faithful to our own nature, hikikomori subjects suffer from environments in which others ignore such ambivalence. The discrepancy between the expectations of others and their own nature is huge and it seems that such expectations must deny their existence. In that context, most hikikomori people continue to blame themselves and experience desperation in their communications with others.

Hikikomori is not just a state of immobility as it has often been represented. Interpreting the hikikomori experience only as immobility obscures the dynamic process of recognizing oneself and confronting ambivalence. In addition, such an interpretation ignores the surroundings of hikikomori subjects, which neither see nor hear their ambivalence. A sociological analysis of the social contexts which tend to ignore the ambivalence in the hikikomori experience is essential to understand the hikikomori experience and the hikikomori problem. Chapter 3 and 5 will examine this issue.

NOTES

1. In Japan, provision of elementary school and junior high-school education is a legal duty, and the administrations of these schools often graduate students even if they have no record of attending school.

2. The majority/minority are Japanese localized English terms that correspond to conventional and unconventional.

3. Arendt here contrasts the public and the private realm and argues that the latter realm lacks appearance and thus a common reality. According to her, modernity has developed the private and intimate realm as never before and "this intensification [of subjective emotions and private feelings in the private life] will always come to pass at the expense of the assurance of the reality of the world and men" (Arendt [1958] 1998, 50). Examining this point in terms of the Japanese family realm may be important, but that is not explored here.

4. Chapter 6 will focus on this process of storytelling about the hikikomori experience.

5. Arendt mentions "the experience of great bodily pain" as "the most private and least communicable of all" (Arendt [1958] 1998, 50–51). However, experience that is difficult to give appearance to, and therefore remains uncertain and private, is not limited to the experience of bodily pain.

Chapter 2

Self-Categorization as Hikikomori

Becoming a Hikikomori Subject

HIKIKOMORI AS A SELF-DEFINITION

The narratives of the hikikomori people in chapter 1 suggest that hikikomori people do not smoothly accept the label hikikomori as a self-definition, but that there is a process of choosing the word "hikikomori" through trial and error. How do people encounter the term "hikikomori," and how do they choose the label as a self-defining category of their own condition and experiences?

Ryōko Ishikawa researched the process of taking on the category of hikikomori (Ishikawa 2007, 107–129). What she focuses on is the process by which "my" experience becomes "our" experience by assuming the category of hikikomori. Many hikikomori subjects say, "I thought I was the only one who was doing this." Having encountered the term "hikikomori," they adopt the label as a self-definition with which they can describe their conditions and experiences. Ishikawa calls such a self-defining category a "vocabulary to express oneself" (*Jiko wo kataru tame no Goi*), and by employing such a vocabulary a person gains access to a wider community of like-minded people (e.g., self-help groups).

However, according to Ishikawa, as they participate in the wider community and thereby acquire interpersonal relationships, the label hikikomori becomes less appropriate, because that term is clearly defined by psychiatrists as "a lack of interpersonal relationships." In fact, a hikikomori subject narrated that he could not consider himself a hikikomori anymore because "when I reflect on my current state in which I can go out, have friends, have interpersonal relationships, I have to wonder if I am in a hikikomori state. No, it's not what it is" (Ishikawa 2007, 108). Thus, Ishikawa concludes the discourse of experts about hikikomori provides hikikomori subjects with a "vocabulary to express oneself," but at the same time it paradoxically deprives hikikomori subjects of the very same vocabulary by defining hikikomori as a lack of interpersonal relationships. This expert definition deprives hikikomori subjects of their vocabulary to express themselves and throws them back "into a state of being nobody" (Ishikawa 2007, 124).

Although Ishikawa's argument is clear, several points still need to be examined. First, Ishikawa's analysis assumes that when hikikomori people cite the experts' discourse as a resource for self-definition, they basically accept the experts' definition without question. However, my interview research (which was done almost a decade after the field research of Ishikawa) suggests that hikikomori subjects do not adopt that expert definition of hikikomori without question as it is in a submissive manner.[1] They integrate the third-personal usage of "hikikomori" in expert discourse with their idiosyncratic usage of that term. We need to clarify what the first-personal meanings and usages of the label "hikikomori" by hikikomori subjects are in detail.

Second, we need to examine how hikikomori subjects choose the label as a self-definition from among various alternatives, especially labels related to mental disorder. The narratives of hikikomori people suggest that there are twists and turns in adopting "hikikomori" over other labels. By examining the process by which a person adopts a self-definition, we will come to understand the first-personal and idiosyncratic meaning of the term "hikikomori."

Therefore, this section focuses on two points: (1) the first-personal uses of the term "hikikomori," which differ from the expert definition, and (2) the process of adopting "hikikomori" as a self-definition. I will focus on the narratives of three interviewees who gave detailed descriptions of their encounters with the term "hikikomori," and three interviewees who shared their thoughts on the relationship between hikikomori and mental disorders.

ENCOUNTERS WITH AND ACCEPTANCE OF THE TERM "HIKIKOMORI"

The Case of Mr. B

Let us take up Mr. B's encounter with the term "hikikomori." He was in a state of withdrawal from the winter of 2001 to the spring of 2003. It was also a period when the mass media were actively reporting on the hikikomori phenomenon. However, he says he did not consider himself a hikikomori at that point.

I was twenty six to twenty eight or twenty nine years old when I was doing nothing. When I think about it now, it is clear that I was in that kind of state as defined by society. In short, there was a period of two to three years when I was doing nothing, neither studying nor looking for a job, and only going to the library and convenience stores. But at that time, I did not think I was a hikikomori. Although it was around the time of the boom in the news and I watched some special programs on hikikomori, I looked down on them, despised those people. I thought I was different from them. It was a strange phenomenon.

Even though he was in a state that could be defined as hikikomori from the third-personal perspective, he did not think of himself as such. How did he come to define himself as hikikomori? He was attracted to the term hikikomori when he saw a TV documentary program about a support group for hikikomori in Sendai city, called "Watage no Kai."

When I saw "Watage no Ie [*sic*]," I felt that the pictures of various people gathering at the place, a private house, seemed to fit in well with me. I think they might have edited in all the good parts of the scenery. There were no strange people. The people who came to the place did not seem sick, so everyone was in harmony, and it was not like they were limping around. It seemed like they were taking a break and looking for the next step or stage. I thought, "Oh, such a place exists," and then I thought, "Let me look for one in Tokyo."

He was fascinated by the way they were "taking a break" and "looking for the next step or stage." At that time, he felt like he was seeking an "escape" rather than a "place to belong to": "I thought that if I could go to such a place, I would be able to be a little more natural even if I were not cured. Well, I did not want to stay at home, so I was searching for a place to escape. It was more of an escape than a place to belong to. It was just painful to stay at home."

When I asked him further about why he felt that "it was painful to stay at home," he replied as follows:

I felt like I was being watched all the time by people around me, or that the people across the street were watching me. I had also become bothered by all sorts of daily life noises. There must have been more outside, but it felt worse when I was alone in my room. I had become hypersensitive; I started to be bothered by noises that would not have bothered me before. When it was worst, I used to jump out of bed at the sound of a newspaper being thrown. Normally I would not notice such things, but [I was startled] even by such a small sound.

Mr. B was deeply stressed out. He attended his grandmother's funeral in the spring of 2003, which was a pivotal moment in his coming to adopt the label "hikikomori." At a relative's house, he was asked "what are you doing for work?" He could not answer anything and just made some awkward gestures. At that point, his younger sister replied, "My brother is helping my father with his work." Mr. B felt a strong inner conflict about this experience:

> I thought, "This is either life or death." I realized for the first time that I was losing my feelings. I was becoming numb. I could not even look at my face and wondered what I looked like. There was a storm in my mind. I only remember picking up the bones of my grandma. I felt like I wanted to go home, but I also did not want to go home. There was a strange contradiction, and I also had a strange idea that maybe my relatives would let me live there because my grandma's place was in the countryside, and I did not know many people there. I thought I should really think about myself when I got home. I was really conflicted.

After the funeral, he returned home feeling very conflicted about his life situation. About a week later, he went to a bookstore and bought a book titled *A Guide to Supporting Hikikomori* (*Hikikomori Shien Gaido*) (Moriguchi, Naura, and Kawaguchi 2002).

> About a week after returning home, I do not remember exactly, I did not have a computer, so I bought a book. I don't know if the book is still sold, but it has a list of support facilities for hikikomori and school refusers throughout Japan. I threw away my pride and bought it. I still remember it. I bought it at the *Bunkyōdō* bookstore in W town. Then, I called a few places. I was very active in that kind of strange way. I made phone calls. At first, I called some place X. But this costed too much, so I decided not to go. I called the Y Club, which I could afford with my own money, but I thought it sounded too heavy. I mean, I thought it seemed for the mentally disordered. So, I said, "I'll visit you just to hear about the place." In the end, I called Z and said, "I would like to ask you about it, but is it okay for someone like me to go?" I lied that I was not hikikomori. I told the person, "I am not doing anything right now, but I am not a pure hikikomori." The staff answered, "Working people can come too. We'll be waiting for you." I do not know who it was, but one of the staff there. I was deeply affected by it. I had not talked to anyone for about two years. Human beings are fragile. You know, they say people who have just come out of hikikomori are moved even by the greeting of the clerk at the convenience store. In the same way, the words "We'll be waiting for you" strangely resonated with me. So, I started going to Z.

Mr. B said he avoided a place that seemed to be "for the mentally disordered." This implies that he imagined some distinction between his status and mental disorders. When I asked if the term "hikikomori" was a key word that led him to purchase the book *A Guide to Supporting Hikikomori*, Mr. B replied as follows:

> I was already aware of it, and I was prepared for it, that I was this [hikikomori]. I thought, "It is not like I have schizophrenia or something." By a process of elimination, I did have some neurosis. I also investigated Morita therapy. I had a bit of obsessive compulsive checking and gaze fear. I thought it might be neurosis, but . . . But I thought, "I do not like Morita therapy." At first, I started by considering it as a mental disorder. I thought it might be obsessive-compulsive disorder. I could not sleep because of the sound of the electric heater or the low-frequency sound. When my condition was worse, the sound of a Japanese foot warmer [*kotatsu*] was almost as bad as the sound of a construction site. I thought, "Maybe there is construction going on outside," so I went out, circled around, and came back home. When I was about to go to bed, I heard a buzzing sound again. I recognized that it was the sound of a *kotatsu*. At that time, before my grandmother died, I thought, "What is going on with me?" So, I went to the library and looked up obsessive-compulsive disorder, Morita therapy, and so on. I thought, "But I do not like these." There were times when I was thinking, "What should I do?" I saw a sign on a telephone pole that said, "Neurosis can be cured," and I was interested in it.

He sought to understand his experience, so he researched mental disorders such as schizophrenia, neurosis, and OCD at the library. He considered whether these mental disorders described his own experience and rejected them one by one, settling on the hikikomori diagnosis by process of elimination:

> I said to myself, "It is not that bad." I read some books on neurosis, and I thought I was kind of okay. I did not get so dominated [by neurotic symptoms]. I thought, "I might be okay." I thought if symptoms got really worse, I would go to a hospital. That was why I kept the phone numbers of hospitals. I used it as a good luck charm. I do not take any sleeping pills now, but I still have it. As a good luck charm. It would be different if I don't have it. I keep it as a good luck charm. I have decided to go to the hospital when things get really bad. When I bought that book [*A Guide to Supporting Hikikomori*], it was not clear, I didn't have it [hikikomori] in my head; however, I think the idea that I might be [a hikikomori] surfaced to my conscious mind. Before that, I thought I had "neurosis." Then, the situation was reversed. I thought I was a hikikomori. A documentary movie was broadcasted on TV at night.[2] There was a documentary

film a younger brother shot about his hikikomori brother, and the making of the documentary was shown. I could not think it was totally unfamiliar to me. Though I hated the elder brother, I thought he was just like me. His feeling of suffering seemed like mine. Gradually, I began to recognize that maybe this is what I look like to others. Until then, I was far away and thought that this was just another group of people, but I started thinking that this was me. And I thought that maybe neurosis was a secondary disorder [of hikikomori]. I wondered which one I should choose. I was not sure about that. I hadn't decided at the time whether I would go to hospital and then go to a support group, or go to a support group and then go to hospital.

He had initially rejected the category of hikikomori, but he gradually came to adopt it as his self-definition. In this process, a pivotal moment was a documentary film that captured the "feeling of suffering" of a hikikomori person. The process of choosing a self-definition was also a process of choosing a course of action between hospitalization and a support group for hikikomori. For Mr. B, purchasing a book on support for hikikomori and actively interpreting his experience according to that category also provided him with an opportunity to connect himself with "society."

Anyway, I was already aware of it when I bought the book [*A Guide to Supporting Hikikomori*]. From there, I tried to heal myself somehow, or rather, to use it as an opportunity. I wanted to use it as a trigger to connect with society, or something less grandiose. Anyway, I wanted to use it as a trigger. I really felt that I was in trouble, so I could not stay at home and get out of it. At that time, I was not thinking about finding a job or becoming an employee, I just wanted to get out and think about it from there. However, I still had a strange pride, so I was still unconvinced.

He understood hikikomori as a category distinct from "mental disorder," and in this respect he follows the usage of psychiatrists who define hikikomori as a "non-psychotic condition." However, he does not totally accept the experts' definition of hikikomori. He identified with the "suffering" of hikikomori subjects in the documentary film, and on that basis gradually came to define himself as hikikomori. He also said that he tried to get a chance to leave the house and to get support by defining himself as a hikikomori subject.

We understand from his narrative that the process by which one comes to define oneself as "hikikomori" takes place in contact with socially available knowledge for self-definition, including a variety of cultural resources such as books, public advertisements and flyers, documentary works, and experts' discourse. The choice of self-definitions is also a choice of self-representation toward others in this context, and it is also connected to the subsequent choices of actions.

The Case of Ms. D

Ms. D was born in the late 1960s. She stopped attending school when she was a sophomore in high school. In her mid-20s, she experienced a state of hikikomori for about two years, and describes how she came to know the term as follows:

> Early in 1997, Mr. Shiokura[3] wrote a series of articles on hikikomori in the morning edition of *Asahi* [the *Asahi Shinbun* newspaper]. When I read it, I thought, "Oh, that is me." . . . I was not school age anymore. At that time, I was in my late twenties. I thought I was a former school non-attendee [*Futōkō*], but I felt it was unreasonable to consider myself as a *Futōkō*. I had been unconnected to school for a long time. It was difficult to think of myself under the category of *Futōkō*, but I still experienced difficulties in my life [*Ikidurasa*]. It was very difficult for me to live. I could not get on well with anyone. When I was thinking about it, I read Mr. Shiokura's newspaper articles and I thought, "Oh, this is just like me." At that time, it was unthinkable for me to work full-time, both physically and mentally. I always thought, "I cannot work, and I don't get on with anyone," throughout my twenties.

"Hikikomori" was a term of self-expression for Ms. D, who had experienced difficulties since dropping out of high school. The following is her answer to my question, "Did you find the term hikikomori as fitting your experience?"

> At first, I thought hikikomori was a very unpleasant term. That feeling lasted for quite a long time. However, I felt that the contents of Shiokura's articles were the same as my experience, that feeling of impossibility to relate with society, though I am curious how I would feel if I read the articles now.

At the time, she was also visiting a clinic, but she never had a clear diagnosis from a doctor.

> I have never been told the diagnosis of my condition, though I guess doctors could have written something if they wanted to. Later, I worked at a clinic and gained some knowledge [of psychiatry]. I still think the only possible diagnosis was an adjustment disorder. . . . They did not even tell me the diagnosis, and I felt like I did not know what the problem was.

What gave her a clue to interpret her experience was the term "hikikomori," which she happened to see in the newspaper article.[4]

> I couldn't categorize myself as anything, but I was clearly having problems. No one could tell me what they were, and I didn't understand them by myself either. In the situation, Shiokura's article gave me the feeling of "this is me." I think there were a lot of people like me at the time. I did not like the term "hikikomori," but it was very effective as a term that could convince me who I was. I felt really relieved by being named.

She was never given a name for the long-lasting difficulties in her life after she dropped out of high school. The term "hikikomori" gave her a clue to interpret and express her own experience of the difficulties in her life. As Ishikawa pointed out, "hikikomori" is "vocabulary to express oneself" that has made it possible for sufferers to describe their experience to others and to connect with others.

Ms. D was later invited to a party to commemorate the publication of Shiokura's book (Shiokura [1999] 2002), which was based on a newspaper series. She met a woman there who told her about a support group for hikikomori people. She joined in the group and became a regular member. For her, encountering the term "hikikomori" became an important step to reconnect with other people.

Other Cases

Mr. B and Ms. D encountered the term "hikikomori" through mass media, like television and newspapers.[5] Other hikikomori people encountered the term "hikikomori" not through the mass media but through interactions with their family, friends, and acquaintances.

A male hikikomori subject, who was born in the early 1970s, spent five years in his late 20s without leaving his house, and communicated with his family only by writing during that period (Sekimizu 2016, 88). To the question "When did you first know the term hikikomori?", he recounted a scene where his father handed him a book borrowed from the library in the late 1990s: Through this event he came to adopt the label.

Another hikikomori person, Mr. E, who was born in the early 1980s, stopped going to school around the end of the first year of junior high. Even after entering high school, he did not actually attend school. Instead, he worked part-time. There were also times when he did not work and stayed mainly at home. When he was 18 years old, his acquaintance told him, "You are a hikikomori."

> I learned the term "hikikomori" when I was 18. An acquaintance told me, "A person like you is called hikikomori," and I took it seriously and I felt depressed.

It sounded a negative image, and it was like being labeled. That was when I started to think of myself as a hikikomori. He was irresponsible because he said to me many years later, "I don't think you are a hikikomori." I thought, "I considered myself so because you said so." I have a tendency to take people's words seriously. When I was in junior high and high school, I did not think of myself as a hikikomori because that concept was probably not widely known at that point.

Mr. E considered hikikomori a negative label attached to him by others, but he eventually accepted the term as a self-definition.

We have looked at several cases of encounters with the label "hikikomori."[6] The knowledge of hikikomori may come through mass media like newspapers and television, or it may be introduced to them in face-to-face interaction. In either case, there is a process of reflecting on their own experience or condition with the term and taking it on as the "vocabulary to express oneself." It is a process of building up the self as a hikikomori subject.

SELF-DEFINITION OF HIKIKOMORI: RELATIONSHIP WITH MENTAL DISORDERS

Mr. B and Ms. D focused on the relationship between the label "hikikomori" and the diagnosis of mental disorders in the process of adopting hikikomori as a self-defining category. Here we discuss in more detail the difference between self-definition using the hikikomori category and using a mental disorder category. Ms. D views hikikomori as different from mental disorder. She interprets the category as an expression of "difficulty in life" (*Ikidurasa*) that is neither disorder nor disability:

It [her difficulty in life] was not a disease, maybe. It was not a disability either. Then, when I wondered what it was, I thought, "Oh, there is a term hikikomori, and there are people like that. This is exactly what I am" and I accepted the term. . . . I think the term "hikikomori" had a kind of power to swallow various things. And it does not mean a disease. It is not a name for a disease or disorder. So, I guess I have no choice but to use it.

She argues that, if hikikomori were a mental disorder, medical treatment would be effective, but *Futōkō* and hikikomori cannot be understood as disorders or disabilities (Field Notes, March 25, 2012).

When the term "hikikomori" is used, [unlike mental disorder categories,] don't you feel that is "not trying to treat the person"? When it comes to treatment-related terms like Morita therapy and AC [Adult Children], they seem to be correcting the person. However, when we use the term "hikikomori," does the word not sound like letting us try not to correct the person, but to change society?

Ms. D gives her own meaning to "hikikomori," which she considers not subject to treatment or correction. Her interpretation of hikikomori agrees with that of many psychiatrists, who define hikikomori as a non-psychotic diagnosis, but her definition is not subordinate to the professional discourse. According to Ms. D, hikikomori is a category that actively refuses psychiatric treatment, implying the need to change society rather than the person.

In contrast to Mr. B and Ms. D, who understand hikikomori as different from mental disorder, some hikikomori subjects believe that mental disorders and hikikomori overlap. Mr. C regards hikikomori as a comprehensive concept that includes illness and disability and, in this way, finds a positive function for it. He has been out of elementary school since the first grade and went to a correspondence high school but dropped out in his second year. After that, he went to a psychosomatic medicine clinic and lived in a state of withdrawal for 10 years before starting a part-time job. Mr. C believes that the concept of hikikomori includes a variety of mental disorders:

> There are probably people with developmental disabilities, people with Asperger [syndrome], people with ADHD [Attention Deficit Hyperactivity Disorder], and so on [inside the category of hikikomori]. There are all kinds of people. But, in the end, they are hikikomori because they cannot integrate well into society. They are trying to find a way through trial and error in the difficulty.

Mr. C sees "hikikomori" as a term that not only overlaps with various mental disorders but also refers to a variety of states of being not well-integrated into society. From this standpoint, he argues that even if a person has a job, if he or she is unable to fit in with society and is going through trial and error, then he or she is in a state of hikikomori. He explains why he interprets hikikomori as such a wide category as follows:

> If someone insists, "This is what a hikikomori is," and if you don't fit into that definition, you have to get out [of the category] again. So, I think it is better to make the category wider. . . . Unless people consider hikikomori widely, some people would think, "I don't fit into this category anymore," and then they have to find another category that does fit. Because there are various characteristics [in each person]. You know, in the end, I am not in a hikikomori state in fact. It is not that I am not working. You know, so right now with doing double work, and to a certain extent, I am earning a certain amount of money. If someone looks at me from the side, he might say, "You are no different from ordinary

people." However, in my mind, I feel that I am certainly different from the ordinary. . . . Then when we talk about what is the goal of hikikomori, it is probably better to say, there might be no goal. I have my own ebbs and flows, and there are times when I cannot move, and when I can.

He says the term "hikikomori" should not have a clear objective definition, but should instead be understood based on each first-personal interpretation, as there is no goal for hikikomori. The category should not be narrowed down. His interpretation of hikikomori is rooted in his recognition of diverse personal characteristics and his own self-understanding as an unfixed being.

His interpretation is not just a way to continue participating in gatherings for hikikomori people. It is also an attempt to redefine the term "hikikomori," which has been defined by experts as a condition to be cured.

When I look at the hikikomori people around me, I see that they have tried and tried again and again, then they arrived at the current life. It is the same for me. I have tried everything, and I have tried to figure out how to make it work. The term "hikikomori" refers to a time when they are unable to adapt to society. The period of hikikomori was the time I realized that my adaptation to society was different from others' and that I couldn't do the same things as everyone else. . . . Even if they [hikikomori people] try to fit in with society, they still cannot do it, so they just try to fit in with themselves, and try to search for the places that fit them. If they only go to places that suit them, there are almost no places for them. Once they know the extent to which they can push themselves, they can see, "I can do this much." . . . The period of trial and error in adapting to society is probably the time of hikikomori. I think it is a time of thinking about what they can do, and how they can do it.

For Mr. C, hikikomori is a label that describes a state of trial and error in adjusting to society. His interpretation of hikikomori is based on his biography where he repeated trial and error and realized what he could do and what he couldn't do to adjust to society.

What, then, does Mr. C think is the relation between hikikomori and mental disorders? When I asked him what he thought about the report (MHLW 2010) by some psychiatrists that most cases of hikikomori entail mental or developmental disorders, he replied as follows:

Some people say that hikikomori is suffering from mental illness or developmental disorders. You know, when I go to a gathering for parents [of hikikomori children], there are a lot of parents trying to manage their [own] anxiety. Then the parents get that kind of [medical] information, and they do not know what kind of hikikomori experience their children have. You know, many parents think they want to do something for their own peace of mind. When I see them,

I think it must be tough [for their children]. . . . You see, I experienced this when I was out of school, and to some extent, my relationship with my parents was [like that]. My parents were looking for relief, and I was being pushed around for it. . . . They say that dealing with the treatment of disorders is enough. So, it is not for the hikikomori subjects but for the third party's relief.

He is concerned that the category of mental disorder—whether assigned by psychiatrists or based on parents' speculation—is used more to reassure parents than for hikikomori subjects' self-understanding. If parents or psychiatrists impose those diagnoses or treatments on hikikomori people, then this makes it more difficult for hikikomori subjects to understand their own experience.

In fact, what he is concerned with is to understand what kind of hikikomori experience they have, in other words, that self-understanding. He repeatedly stresses the importance of finding a category that promotes self-understanding. For Mr. C, adopting the self-definition of hikikomori is a way to advance his self-understanding and explain himself to others. Whether anxiety disorder, developmental disorder, or hikikomori, the more options they have in their vocabulary for describing themselves, the better.

Finally, let us examine the case of Minoru Katsuyama. He was born in 1971 and has been living as a hikikomori subject for 20 years, since dropping out of high school. He has published two books (Katsuyama 2001, 2011) about his experience as and thoughts on hikikomori, while writing a blog about his daily life and advocacy. When I asked about the relationship between mental disorder and hikikomori, he replied as follows:

Mental disorder and hikikomori are both home ground for me. I know there are people who are proud of the idea that hikikomori is not a mental illness, but I think I can find a compromise with such people. . . . Hikikomori is the most relevant problem for me. It stands out the most. As a mentally disabled person, I am not very interesting. I cannot even hear auditory hallucinations, and I fall behind the people of "Bethel House" [*Beteru no Ie*].[7] I cannot make anyone laugh when I say, "The rainy season makes me feel gloomy, but I can manage my mood with antidepressants." As a disabled person, I have no strong point. I cannot stand on the stage. I am one of the many people and I am of low ranking. In the field of hikikomori, I am a "master" [*Meijin*]. But that is for the people around me to decide.

He can talk about himself with the terms of mental disorder, but within that category, he is just "one of the many." He has clearly chosen hikikomori as his self-definition. One of the reasons for this is that he thinks that hikikomori has a connotation that is difficult to capture with other terms:

Hikikomori is the one that fits me best. I have a feeling that NEETs might start working. NEETs want to work, but they cannot. Hikikomori people don't work because they don't want to, which sounds very selfish, so they keep their true feelings to themselves. This is modesty. In a way this is the heart of literature or poetry. Researchers need to understand this gentle heart.

He subjectively chooses the label "hikikomori" as a self-definition. "Hikikomori" is a term to express his way of life.[8]

Each hikikomori subject interprets the term "hikikomori" in their own unique way, regardless of whether they consider hikikomori to be nonpsychotic or not. None of their interpretations are totally subordinate to the professional discourse. For Ms. D, hikikomori implies that it would be better to change society, not the individual. For Mr. C, hikikomori means "trial and error in adapting to society." For Katsuyama "hikikomori" is a word to describe his policy of life.

Based on the work of M. Foucault (Foucault 1976), the philosopher of science Ian Hacking focused on the process in which people classified by expert-crafted categories of "human kinds" start to have their own voice.[9] They argue they are not just objects to be named, classified, and studied by experts, but that they are subjects who have idiosyncratic knowledge of themselves. The "human kinds" from which such a subjective point of view emerges are specifically understood a "self-ascriptive category" (Hacking 1996, 380–382).

Hikikomori subjects have developed hikikomori as a self-ascriptive category in Hacking's sense. Hikikomori people such as Mr. C, Ms. D, and Katsuyama have ceased to be objects to be defined and categorized by experts and have become subjects who generate knowledge about themselves.[10]

BECOMING A HIKIKOMORI SUBJECT: NOT SUBORDINATION TO THE CATEGORY

As Mr. C and Ms. D's interpretation of hikikomori clearly displayed, hikikomori subjects attach their unique meanings of the category to fit their own experiences. Adopting a category as a self-description does not mean subordinating oneself to a third-personal definition of the category. In other words, accepting a category as self-descriptive is a process of rejecting, at least in part, the objective (third-personal) meaning assigned to the category, and reinterpreting it by oneself, incorporating into it one's own subjective (first-personal) meaning.

We are forced to describe and define our experiences in the context of the socially available knowledge in our biographically determined situations. This knowledge is not something of our own individual creation. However, our self-definitions are not unilaterally determined by socially available knowledge, or third-personal definitions based on that; they also represent our interpretation of that knowledge and our negotiation with objective (third-personal) and subjective (first-personal) definitions.[11]

CONCLUSION

Ishikawa observed that the hikikomori category as defined by experts becomes useless as a "vocabulary to express oneself" when hikikomori people regain interpersonal relationships. This is a dilemma for them. However, some hikikomori people continue to use the term as a resource for their self-description. They redefine it in a way that better expresses their own understanding of their states and experiences, a way that doesn't preclude the possibility of forming interpersonal relationships. This process of reinterpreting "hikikomori" will be discussed again in chapter 6.

NOTES

1. The hikikomori research analyzed in Ishikawa (2007) was conducted in the first half of the 2000s. Looking back on the early 2000s, she reflects, "When I started the survey 12 years ago, there was almost no active expression from the hikikomori people. That is why I started the survey, because I wanted to hear what the people had to say. Now, I think there are people who are willing to share their stories, and there seems to be an atmosphere that accepts them" (Field Notes, March 23, 2013). In other words, the circulated narratives about hikikomori at that time were mostly the third-personal, and the first-personal usage that countered the expert definition had not yet clearly emerged. Ishikawa also noted the use of novel categories like "ex-hikikomori" and "OBs," but she didn't discuss them (Ishikawa 2007, Chap. 4).

2. This refers to the documentary film "Home" directed by Takahiro Kobayashi, which was released in 2001.

3. Yutaka Shiokura is a journalist for the *Asahi Shinbun* newspaper. In 1997, he began a series of articles on hikikomori in the *Asahi Shinbun*.

4. Until the early 1990s, the term "hikikomori" was not widely known, and there were many people like Ms. D who were forced to live mainly at home, but without being labeled and without being able to find self-definitions of their experiences.

5. In Ishikawa's interviews, a man born in 1973 came to know the term "hikikomori" from the psychiatrist Tamaki Saitō's website in the late 1990s. A woman born in 1977 says that she "learned that she was a hikikomori" after watching a TV program featuring Tamaki Saitō around 2000 (Ishikawa 2007, 119–122). These cases show the influence of the mass media, especially the influence of statements by Saitō, who had been vigorously raising awareness of the problem of hikikomori through the mass media since the late 1990s.

6. Interviewees examined here remembered encountering the term "hikikomori." However, a hikikomori person born in the late 1980s said that she did not remember her first encounter with the term "hikikomori." Yet it is natural that she would not remember that if the word had already widely circulated and become a common word when she grew up (Sekimizu 2016, 105).

7. A community and activity center for people with mental disorders, located in Urakawa-chō, Hokkaido, Northern Japan. It started in 1984 and is known for its unique activities for people with mental disorders (Nakamura 2013).

8. However, Katsuyama does not deny that he chooses the mental disorder category as a self-definition. Speaking of his own diagnostic category, depression, Katsuyama says, "I thought everyone who went to a psychiatrist was crazy. . . . It was hard for me if what I thought was literature and beliefs turned out to be symptoms of illness according to a diagnosis. I thought I would have to give up all my beliefs and stuff. However, depression also has beliefs and philosophies."

9. Hacking also points out that categories that originally represented human status or behaviors are diverted into categories that represent human classification (Hacking 1996). Hikikomori was also originally a category to describe a state or behavior of humans. The title of the book *Hey, Hikikomori. It is time to go outside*, published in 1997 (Kudō 1997), indicates that this term was already used in that way by that year at the latest.

10. Hacking focuses on the process of "making up people," and points out that there are two opposite vectors: labeling by the expert community versus the autonomous activities of labeled people (Hacking 2002, Chap. 6).

11. Schutz focuses on the case where a category is unilaterally imposed on people who do not intend to define themselves in that way. He wrote: "But if he is compelled to identify himself as a whole with that particular trait or characteristic which places him in terms of the imposed system of heterogeneous relevances into a social category he had never included as a relevant one in the definition of his private situation, then he feels that he is no longer treated as a human being in his own right and freedom, but is degraded to an interchangeable specimen of the typified class. He is alienated from himself, a mere representative of the typified traits and characteristics. He is deprived of his right to the pursuit of happiness" (Schutz [1957] 1964, 256–257).

Chapter 3

Hikikomori as a Japanese Social Problem

Focusing on Families with Hikikomori Children

THE HIKIKOMORI PROBLEM FOR FAMILIES

This chapter examines the hikikomori problem for families with hikikomori children. Interestingly, families are not necessarily concerned about their children's habit of staying home. A survey published in 2010 (KHJ 2010) by a nonprofit organization, the KHJ National Association of Families with Hikikomori (*KHJ Zenkoku Hikikomori Kazokukai Rengōkai*) (KHJ),[1] asked family members (mostly parents) about the "degree of hikikomori" of their children.[2]

Figure 3.1 shows the results: 15.7% of the respondents answered that their hikikomori family member "participates in socializing with friends and community activities," and 50.9% answered that they "do not get involved with others but do go out." The respondence indicates that nearly 70% of the hikikomori subjects go out. Only about 20% of the subjects "do not go out," and of these, only about 3% "stay in their room." The KHJ 2016 survey report shows that, to the question of whether the hikikomori subject "goes out freely," 35% answered "strongly agree," and 33% answered "agree." This result, with 68% answering that the hikikomori subjects could go out relatively freely, is equally surprising (KHJ 2016, 10). The 2020 survey report also shows similar results: 29.8% chose "strongly agree," and 26.6% chose "agree" to the question of whether "the hikikomori subject can go out freely" (KHJ 2020, 31).

Although the respondents' children may have experienced periods in the past when they did not go out, the current condition of the majority of hikikomori children is that they go out—at least spatially—and are not shut-in. Thus, for parents, "hikikomori" cases do not always mean those who

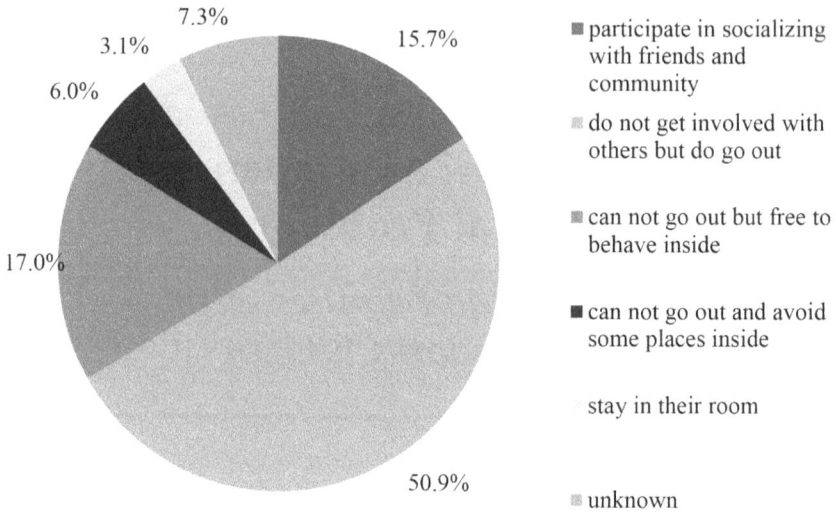

Figure 3.1   The Degree of Hikikomori. *Source*: Created by the author based on data from KHJ (2010).

stay in their room and do not leave home despite the word's original meaning "withdrawal."

These results show that the core of the hikikomori problem for families is not the withdrawn behaviors or withdrawn conditions of their hikikomori family members. So then, what is the core of the hikikomori problem for families, specifically parents?

In 2008, the Tokyo Metropolitan Government conducted a survey of parents with hikikomori children in Tokyo, titled *Fact-finding Survey on Hikikomori: Withdrawn Youth and Family Concerns* (Tokyo Metropolitan Youth and Public Safety Headquarters 2009).[3] The number of valid responses was 185.

This survey asked about family difficulties with the following query: "We guess you must have burdens as a family [with hikikomori people]. Thinking about the past few months, to what extent have you experienced the following?"

The results were as follows: (1) "Anxiety regarding life in my old-age" had the most common response with 90.3%, including "strongly agree" (62.2%) and "agree" (28.1%). (2) "Worries about [the hikikomori subject's] siblings' lives and future" had a total response of 82.8% (51.4% "strongly agree" and 31.4% "agree"). (3) "The financial burden related to the hikikomori subject is heavy" had 70.8% affirmation (25.4% "strongly agree" and 45.4% "agree") (Tokyo Metropolitan Youth and Public Safety Headquarters 2009, 78–79) (figure 3.2).[4]

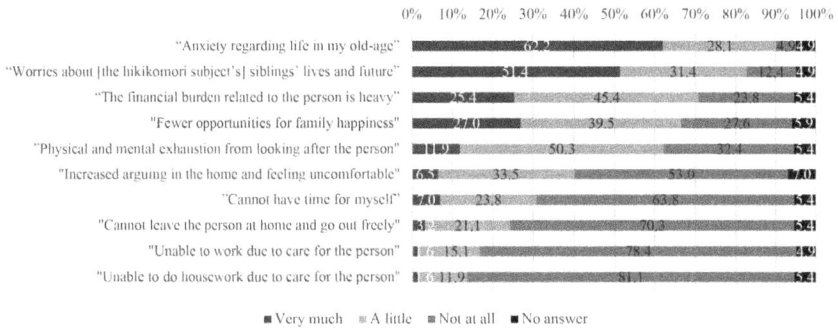

Figure 3.2 **About Family Difficulties.** *Source*: Created by the author based on data from Tokyo Metropolitan Youth and Public Safety Headquarters (2009).

These results suggest that the core of the hikikomori problem for families is anxiety about the family's future. However, this survey does not provide any more concrete information on the details of their anxiety. Therefore, it is necessary to go back to the surveys of the KHJ Family Association to confirm the nature of this anxiety about the family's future. In the KHJ survey report "Support Needs for the 'Hikikomori Community Support Center (tentative name)'" released in 2009 (KHJ 2009), the following comments are from families (specifically parents).

> If they [the hikikomori children] do not work and earn a living, parental resources could be exhausted. In the current economic and employment scenario, it seems that there is no job for them. Please find work for hikikomori people that they can engage in.

> It is easy to say, "I just hope for them to live." However, the day we die, their "living" is at stake. In that situation, I hope there is at least one system that guarantees their "living."

Another KHJ report also contains statements from respondents that elucidate the needs and anxieties of parents with hikikomori children. (KHJ 2016, 79–80)

> I think their own national pension is not enough for my child to live on, so I, as a parent, pay for their National Pension Fund. I do not want other siblings to be involved in financial trouble, so I, as a parent, work as much as I can and [provide financial security] for my hikikomori child, but I am anxious. I imagine that it would be nice if there could be a self-sufficient life where hikikomori people can live [together] in a kind of group home, cultivating the fields, growing crops, and living off the pension[.]

Currently, my child lives with us, parents and family, and we parents work so
that we could live normally. However, [our] retirement is approaching, so I am
worried about what would happen when our income decreases.

I have hoped and tried hard to enable them to live by themselves. However, the
reality is harsh. I have only anxieties. . . . There must be many children who
cannot go out. If someone can help us with their future lives, we will be relieved.
I promise to continue to do my best as a parent so that they can live without
assistance from others.

Parents with hikikomori children express intense anxiety about their family
life in the future, and they especially express anxiety about their children's
lives after the parents' death.

These descriptions suggest that the anxiety over the life security of the
family unit—and not the distinctively withdrawn condition of hikikomori
children—is the real core of the hikikomori problem for families. The
Tokyo Metropolitan Government survey also suggests the anxiety at issue is
specifically anxiety about the life security for all family members, including
parents, hikikomori children, and their siblings.

However, why do families with hikikomori adult children—who can often
"leave home freely" and whose average age is in their 30s[5]—continue to
worry about their life security as a family unit even after their hikikomori
children reach adulthood? Why are families unable to find other life security
entities for their adult hikikomori children? Why do the jobless adult children
continue to be excluded from the labor market, public assistance, and other
forms of life security and instead keep relying on their families? These are
the questions that need to be answered.

These questions require exploring the Japanese life security system,
which causes and maintains the hikikomori problem as anxiety about the
sustainability of family life with hikikomori children. This chapter explores
how Japanese society provides life security for hikikomori children and
also how it excludes them from life security. More precisely, this chapter
considers life security systems as a social structural background for the
hikikomori problem, which imposes the life security anxiety on families with
hikikomori children.[6]

PERSPECTIVES OF ANALYSIS: MARKET, GOVERNMENT, AND FAMILY AS ACTORS OF LIFE SECURITY

What approach is feasible to the Japanese life security system (*seikatsu hoshō
sisutemu*)? Life security sounds like a vague concept. As labor economist

Mari Ōsawa puts it, "In order to live, people at least require (have needs for) goods such as food, clothing, and housing, as well as services such as care during childhood and illness" (Ōsawa 2013, 48). The scope of life security is comprehensive, ranging from housing and medical care to nursing care services, all of which satisfy people's basic needs.

This chapter focuses on three main providers of basic needs and their relationship. We can identify the following three major social systems that have primary importance for the provision of life security. The first is the market, the second is the government (public sector), and the third is the family (figure 3.3).

This analytical framework follows Esping-Andersen's theory of welfare regimes. According to him, "Welfare regimes must be identified much more systematically in terms of the inter-causal triad of state, market, and family" (Esping-Andersen 1999, 35). These three inter-related poles constitute a life security system that provides the welfare of people. He typified this tripolar system of welfare production into three types: *conservative regime*, *social democratic regime*, and *liberal regime*.[7] However, the focus of this chapter is not on an exploration of the typology of welfare regimes or an international comparison of them, but on recasting the hikikomori problem for families using the framework of this tripolar system.

Each of the three systems, in general, works as an essential provider of welfare. A basic form of life security in the market is the commodification of goods and services. In the market system, people attain goods and services as commodities with money. Workers also commodify themselves as labor power in the labor market. The wage as payment is a vital welfare resource that provides money and guarantees laborers' livelihoods.

However, "labor-power-as-a-commodity" is another name for the worker. Such a commodity is called a "fictitious commodity"—a category which

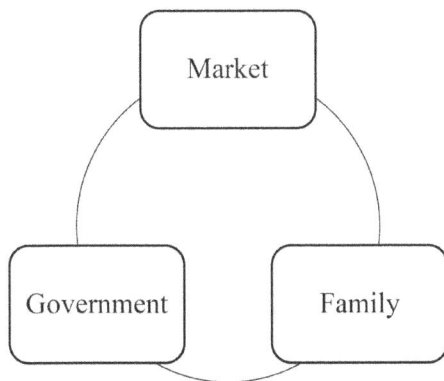

Figure 3.3   Three Basic Providers of Life Security. *Source*: Created by the author.

includes workers, nature, and money, for all of them are not produced as commodities, and the market cannot treat them in the same way as usual commodities (Polanyi 1944). The wage for the labor commodity cannot be determined only by the balance between supply and demand in the market. Wages cannot be pure market prices but are legally regulated. In the course of the long-lasting struggle between employers and employees, a legal agreement of a "fair price" and a "fair treatment" for labor has been established. The minimum wage and restrictions on working hours protect the worker's life as a "fictitious commodity." These regulations are essential to workers' life sustainability, which the self-adjustment mechanism of the market would destroy.

The second system, the government,[8] provides life security in the form of de-commodification. In unemployment, aging, or disabilities, the government redistributes money, goods, and services in the form of public benefits or pensions. In addition to these benefits, legal regulations such as taxation and the minimum wage can also be regarded as the governmental life security system (Takegawa 2007, 6). This life security provision is usually called "social security." This life security through the social security system is called *de-commodification*, because social security guarantees a living independently from the labor market.[9]

The third system of welfare production is the family. The family provides life security not through commodification in the market nor de-commodification by the government but rather by "pre-commodification" of family members in family units (Esping-Andersen 1990, 38–41). Life security in the family unit includes the provision of goods such as food, clothing, housing, and physical and mental care based on family membership. The pre-commodification of the family remains an essential part of the life security system, especially in less-developed welfare states such as Japan and southern European countries (Italy, Greece, Spain, and Portugal) (Uzuhashi 2011, Chap. 2).

This chapter aims to clarify how the three primary inter-determinant systems result in Japanese family anxiety about the life security of hikikomori children. First, concerning the market, the following processes will be examined: (1) how the labor market became a significant part of the life security system in Japanese society including the development of life security by private corporations during the 1950s–1980s, and (2) the changes of the private corporate life security function after the 1990s. Second, regarding the government, the following aspects of Japanese social security system will be examined: (1) characteristics of the social security system in postwar Japan and the benefits for disabled people, and (2) education as a support for commodification. Third, with regard to the family, the following characteristics will be examined: (1) the historical role of life security played by the family, including how the family's obligation to support immature children is legally defined, and (2) the absence of public intervention in family issues.

LIFE SECURITY THROUGH THE LABOR MARKET: COMMODIFICATION

Development of Life Security through the Labor Market

This section examines the role of life security through the labor market in postwar Japanese society. Life security by the labor market has grown throughout the postwar period. Figure 3.4 shows the ratio of "Self-employed workers," "Family workers," and "Employees" to the total working population.

The number of employed workers signifies the tendency of the commodification of labor power. In 1953, the self-employed (mainly in agriculture) and their family member workers accounted for nearly 60% of all workers. However, since then, the ratio of the self-employed worker has decreased, and instead, the employee has been consistently increasing.

From an international perspective, the spread of the commodification of labor power in Japan had been slow. The majority of workers, 56.5%, were self-employed and family workers in 1955, the year Japan's rapid economic growth started, compared to 18.0% in the United States and 24.3% in West

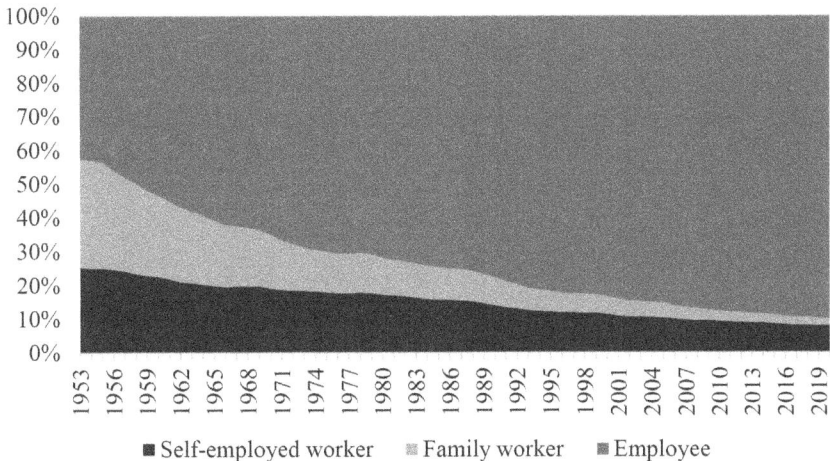

Figure 3.4 Ratio of Workers by Status in Employment. *Source*: Created by the author based on data from the Historical data 4 (1) of the Labour Force Survey. https://www.stat.go.jp/data/roudou/longtime/03roudou.html.

Germany in 1957 (Nomura 2014, 212).[10] Japan was a "semi-agricultural country," where half of the workers engaged in the primary industry before high economic growth in 1950 (Yoshikawa 2012, 21).

Japanese society has changed dramatically from a semi-agricultural society to an employee-majority society after World War II. The percentage of self-employed and family workers has continued to decline, having fallen below 50% in 1959. In its stead, the number of "commodified" employees who receive wages has increased, reaching 89.5% of the labor force in 2020.[11]

During the period of rapid economic growth, large corporations took on responsibility for the life security of their employees. A typical form of this is the "living wage" model as an embodiment of the "family wage" concept, in which the earnings of a husband are supposed to support the whole family (Kimoto 2004, 304–305). The Japan Electrical Industry Trade Union Council initially demanded this wage model, and it was realized early in the postwar period. This wage model spread widely to other industries. The characteristic of this wage model is that the living wage, which accounts for 80% of the total wage, is "calculated according to the worker's age and the number of family members" (Kimoto 2003, 304). In addition to this living wage model, a wide variety of "corporate welfare" programs for employees were introduced and developed, mainly by large corporations; family allowances supporting childcare and child education, corporate pensions, housing benefits, company housing, hospital facilities, recreational facilities, and low-interest home loans.[12]

Employees demanded that corporations, not the government, guarantee their life security and that of their families.[13] These demands on corporate welfare contrast with Western European countries, where employees aimed to enhance the life security system through expansion of the welfare state by supporting labor parties (Gotō 2004).[14]

Many large corporations introduced home loans for their employees in order to make "it possible for young full-time employees to acquire their own houses by lending them housing loans with low interest," and at the same time "made them even more dependent on the company for the loan repayment" (Watanabe 2004, 44).

However, political scientist Osamu Watanabe points out that the proportion of employees working for large corporations was not a majority of the total workforce. For example, in 1970, the ratio of employees in large corporations accounted for only about 13% of the total labor force and 20% of all employees. Despite the small number of employees who enjoyed a high level of life security from companies, the consciousness of "corporate society" expanded even to employees in small and medium-sized corporations as well as the public sector. The prevailing belief was that living standards would improve through corporate prosperity and economic growth and that corporations are responsible for the life security of employees. Even workers in small and medium-sized enterprises expected increases in their wages and a narrowed gap with major corporations under the high economic growth. This expectation was also shared in the public sector, because the public-sector wage was linked to the private-sector wage (Watanabe 2004, 49–51).

As employees' expectations for life security provided by the private corporate sector (in lieu of the public social security system) grew, employees became even more loyal to their corporate employers. The labor laws scholar Keiichiro Hamaguchi analyzes the merits and demerits of the living wage in companies as follows: employees tend to continue working for the same company because they receive a living wage commensurate with age, and thus the incentive to change jobs is significantly lost. At the same time, employees remain loyal to their corporate employers to minimize the risk of bankruptcy or dismissal (Hamaguchi 2009, 121–126).[15]

Mari Ōsawa characterizes the life security provided by private corporations as a "male-breadwinner" model. This life security model assumes the gender role division of labor in which males as full-time employees earn a living wage for their families, while females as housewives engage in housework and provide care for family members (Ōsawa 2007). Female full-time employees were under the marriage retirement system, which forced them to retire when they got married. A discriminatory retirement age system and a discriminatory promotion system were also imposed on female workers (Watanabe 2004, 44–45).[16]

This private corporate life security model rapidly expanded during high economic growth, despite various problems such as gender inequality, inequality of the extent of life security between corporations, disparity between full-time and part-time employees, and excessive loyalty to corporations. As shown in figure 3.5, the unemployment rate in Japan was around 2% from the 1950s to the 1970s. Until 1995, the unemployment rate remained lower than 3%. The life security system provided by private corporations and the public subsidies covered almost all workers.

Although the cabinet led by Kakuei Tanaka positioned 1973 as the "first year of social welfare" and worked on establishing welfare-state measures like free medical care for the elderly and pension system reform, the government shifted the policy direction to the "Japanese-style of welfare society" theory (*Nihon-gata Fukushi Shakai Ron*) after the oil crisis in the fall of the same year. This policy emphasized the private corporation and the family as the primary foundation of welfare for Japanese population. The limited level of the government's social security made people even more dependent on corporate welfare (Kimoto 2004, 310–311).

Through 1980s, Japanese government tried to reinforce and maintain the Japanese style of welfare society. Economic growth slowed to around 4%

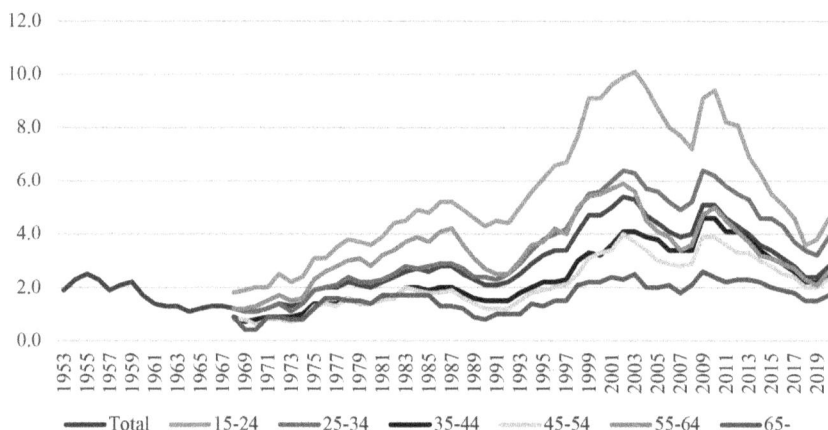

Figure 3.5 Unemployment Rate by Age Group (10-Year Age Group). *Source*: Created by the author based on data from the Historical data 3 (9) of the Labour Force Survey. https://www.stat.go.jp/data/roudou/longtime/03roudou.html.

per year on average after the mid-1970s, and the shadow of job insecurity loomed. However, corporate welfare and family welfare were emphasized over government welfare by the Japanese-style welfare society policy. For employees, "it became more important to demonstrate loyalty to the company," and the term "company-centered man" (*Kaisha-Ningen*) enter the lexicon in the 1970s (Kimoto 2004, 310). This pressure is a social background of Kazuki Ueyama's fear to be a full-time employee mentioned in chapter 1.

Decline of Life Security through the Labor Market

From the 1990s, Japan entered a phase of a decline in life security provided by the labor market. The unemployment rate rose rapidly, reaching 5.6% in 2000. The unemployment rate among the younger generation between the ages of 15 and 24 became exceptionally high, reaching a record of 10.1% in 2003 (figure 3.5). Secure employment has become an acute problem for the younger generation.

The ratio of non-regular employment also increased through the 1990s and the 2000s. The percentage of non-regular employment was 15.3% of the total employed population in 1984, but it exceeded 30% in 2002. The percentage of males was 7.7% in 1984; it exceeded 10% in 1997; and it was over 20% for the first time in 2008. That of females rose from 29.0% in 1984 to 53.5% in 2008.[17]

The rate of non-regular employment is also particularly high among the younger age groups: 26.0% of males aged 15–24 (excluding those still in school) were non-regular employee as of 2002; for men aged 25–34, the rate was 3.3% in 1988 and exceeded 10% in 2003; for those aged 35–44, the rate was from 3.0% in 1988 to 6.2% in 2004, more than doubled (figure 3.6). For women, 35.0% of women aged 15–24 (excluding those still in school) were non-regular employee in 2002; for women aged 25–34, the figure was 25.9% in 1988 and 37.7% in 2003; and for those aged 35–44, the figure was 47.6% in 1988 and 55.6% in 2004 (figure 3.7). On the contrary, the number of young full-time employees who could gain traditional life security from

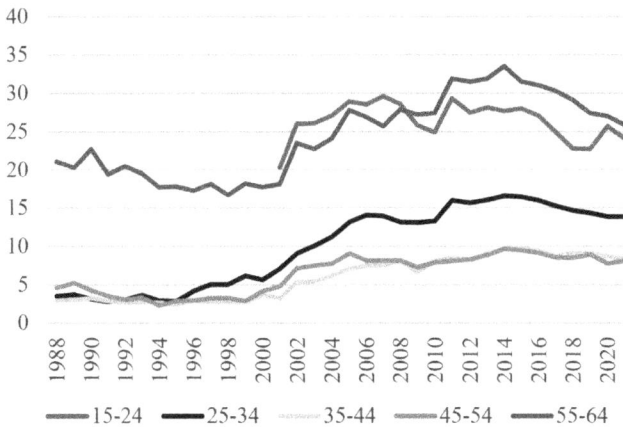

Figure 3.6 Rates of Non-Regular Employee (Male, 10-Year Age Group). *Source*: Created by the author based on data from the Historical data 9 (1) of the Labour Force Survey.https://www.stat.go.jp/data/roudou/longtime/03roudou.html.

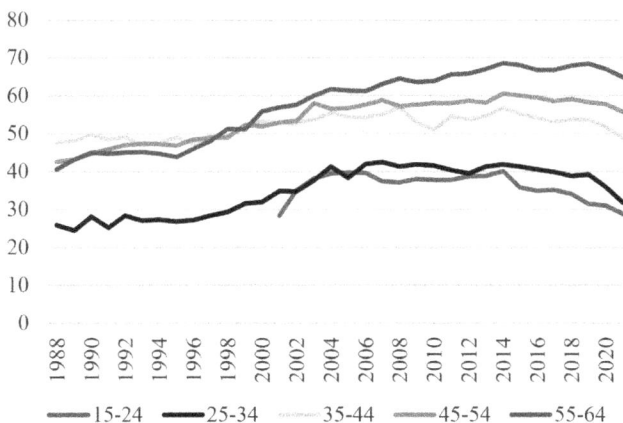

Figure 3.7 Rates of Non-Regular Employee (Female, 10-Year Age Group). *Source*: Created by the author based on data from the Historical data 9 (1) of the Labour Force Survey.https://www.stat.go.jp/data/roudou/longtime/03roudou.html.

their companies decreased.[18] The originally high rate of part-time employ-ment among females indicates that the female labor force has been regarded as household auxiliary labor under the male-breadwinner model.

Although the rising unemployment rate and the ratio of non-regular employment suggest a decrease in young employees who could gain access to stable corporate life security, people did not realize the problem until the mid-2000s. Labor law scholar Keiichiro Hamaguchi observes:

> From the present point of view, the following is almost universally recognized: It was the 1990s when the young people "who could get jobs without doubt, even if not everyone could find a job for which they hoped" began to be excluded from the full-time employment system that they were supposed to be included in and were forced to take the path of low-wage, precarious non-regular workers known as "Freeters." However, this recognition was not established until the mid-2000s. (Hamaguchi 2013a, 151)

People criticized the younger generation who failed to find full-time jobs as being "immature in work consciousness" and "indulgently dependent on others" (*amae*) in the 1990s (Hamaguchi 2013a, 151–160).

One of the reasons for this rapid increase in unemployment and non-regular employment was the deregulation of the labor market, which was inaugurated by the manifesto of the Japan Federation of Employers' Associations (*Nihon Keieisha Dantai Renmei*), "Japanese-style Management for a New Era," published in 1995. This manifesto announced a need to change "Japanese employment practices," including lifetime employment practice and seniority-based wages, and it also proposed a policy to make employment more flexible—expanding non-regular employment. Subsequently, the Liberal Democratic Party amended the Labor Standard Law and the Worker Dispatching Law and promoted the deregulation and liquidation of the labor market (cf. An, Lin, and Shinkawa 2015, 15–16). The series of labor law reforms means that the government approved the curtailing of corporate welfare, which is the cornerstone of the Japanese-style welfare society policy.

What has occurred in the labor market since the 1990s is an increase in the number of people excluded from the life security measures provided by private corporations by falling into non-regular employment or unemployment. The increase is particularly marked among members of the younger generation, many of whom find it difficult to become to be included in for life security by private companies and are forced to continue living with their parents. As chapter 4 will examine, the Japanese government established "youth independence" as political issue after the 2000s.

A governmental report from the fiscal year 2013 showed a rise in unmarried people living with their parents in the 20s and 30s age groups. Those who were single and living with their parents increased from 1995 to 2010 as follows: from 52.4% to 53.1% of those in their 20s, from 18.8% to 27.6% of those 30–34, and from 10.9% to 20.1% of those 35–39. The 35–39 age group increased significantly. The number of people living with their parents into their 30s increased from around 850,000 to 1,930,000. The rate of living with parents is higher among those with unstable employment (Ministry of Land, Infrastructure, Transport and Tourism 2013, 33–34).

At the same time, corporate welfare for full-time employees, which had replaced the governmental life security provisions, was also reduced. For example, corporate pensions were reduced or abolished. An, Lin, and Shinkawa show that "the number of qualified pension plans, which had been the core of corporate pensions, were dissolved one after another after 1993, and decreased by about 20,000 by the turn of the twenty-first century" (An, Lin, and Shinkawa 2015, 15).

During rapid economic growth, Japanese corporations sought to provide life security for their employees and their families in place of the welfare state. However, it has transformed drastically since the 1990s. The same corporations tend to regard employees just as personnel costs during economic stagnation. Since then, the life security measures provided by companies for full-time employees has diminished, thus the corporate welfare system has excluded an increasing number of people, especially among the younger generation.

Changes in the Quality of the Labor Market

The industrial structure (i.e., the structural composition of industry) also transformed dramatically after the end of high economic growth in Japan. According to the national census, the number of workers in primary industry (agriculture, forestry, and fisheries) has been consistently decreasing, except for the period immediately after the end of World War II. It accounted for about 3.2% of the workforce in 2020. Secondary industries (construction and manufacturing industries) have also declined since their peak in the 1970s. On the other hand, the tertiary sector (various service industries) is consistently increasing: 73.8% of workers were in tertiary industries in 2020 (figure 3.8).[19]

The transformation of the industrial structure meant the labor market became exclusive of a particular segment of the populace searching for regular employment. Sociologist Yukimitsu Nishimura writes the following at the beginning of his article dealing with the transitional changes for youth: "Modern Japanese society is shifting the weight of employment from the manufacturing industry to the service industry. The contemporary workers' skills required today are not

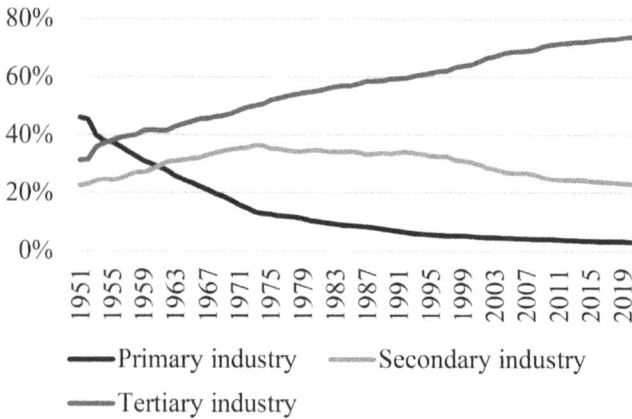

Figure 3.8 Percentage of Workers by Industry. *Source*: Created by the author based on data from the Japan Institute for Labour Policy and Training (Figure 4-1 "Number of Workers by Industry").https://www.jil.go.jp/kokunai/statistics/timeseries/html/g0204.html.

limited to so-called 'craftsmanship' [*monozukuri*] in factories, . . . but people are required to be involved in the production and the provision of a variety of interpersonal services and communication" (Nishimura 2014, 384).

This transformation of the industrial structure led to a change of required skills in the labor market, so job seekers who lack the skills necessary for "the production and provision of various interpersonal services and communication" now have trouble finding jobs. In other words, this specific type of person, who is considered not sociable enough, tends to experience difficulty getting stable employment and thus tends to be excluded from the life security measures provided by corporate welfare.

LIFE SECURITY THROUGH THE
GOVERNMENT: DE-COMMODIFICATION

Characteristics of the Social Security System in Postwar Japan

As we have already seen, governmental life security in postwar Japanese society did not sufficiently develop because Japanese society supposed private corporations and family should provide the base of life security for employees and their families. As a result, the life security provisions for the working-age population from the social security system essentially remain at a low level.

Social policy scholar Takafumi Uzuhashi lists the following four characteristics of the Japanese social security system compared to other

OECD countries: (1) the legal minimum wage is lower and the receipt period for unemployment insurance is shorter than the OECD average; (2) public assistance is one of the most comprehensive and systematic among the OECD countries, but the number of recipients is small; (3) social benefits for the working poor, such as housing benefits, are underdeveloped; and (4) tax credits for low-income groups have not been introduced (Uzuhashi 2011, 143–147).

According to Uzuhashi, these facts are because the Japanese social security system lacks an important layer of social security: social benefits. They are benefits for daily living needs and are financed by public funds, which include medical assistance, housing benefits, child benefits, and family benefits, and differ from social insurance in that they do not require advance contributions. The safety nets in Japanese society consist of a first layer of "employment," a second of "social insurance," and a third of "public assistance"—but it has not developed any "social benefits" (social allowance) between the second and third layers (Uzuhashi 2011, Chap. 7). As previous sections examined, the Japanese style of welfare society policy assumed that private corporations and individual families should handle these functions of social benefits.

In contrast, many OECD countries have introduced social benefits (social allowance) as a system that plays an essential role in the life security function of the welfare state (Uzuhashi 2011, 143–147). According to housing policy researcher Yōsuke Hirayama, the percentage of households receiving housing allowances is 23% in France, 20% in Sweden, and 14% in the Netherlands, while in Japan, there is almost no public housing allowance system (Hirayama 2011, 17–18).[20]

Although the Japanese social security system positions public assistance as the last safety net, which also includes housing benefits, there are administrative hurdles as well as an extreme stigma to receiving such assistance. Asset requirements are rigorous, such as the requirement that savings be less than half a month's worth of minimum living expenses (Gotō 2012, 153). The social stigma is reinforced by the Japanese government's assumption that the life security for the working-age population should be provided by private corporations and families as much as possible. As a result, it is difficult for people to have stable housing independent of their families (parents) unless they land full-fledged jobs and are subsequently included in the corporate welfare system. This private-sector-dependent social security system constitutes a social background of the anxiety of hikikomori subjects and their families for their life security.

Low Benefits in the Field of Disability

What about the life security for those publicly recognized as having difficulties working, namely disabled people? By international comparison, the number of recipients of disability benefits in Japan and the scale of cash benefits are both low. The relatively small number of disability benefits recipients is evident in the OECD report. Figure 3.9 shows the ratio of disability beneficiaries to the population aged 20–64 years old in 31 OECD countries (note the data is from 2012 or else the latest year available) (OECD 2016, 32).[21] While the OECD average for disability beneficiaries is about 6.0% of the working-age population, it is 2.1% in Japan, the third-lowest after Mexico and South Korea. These data suggest that the range of those eligible to receive disability benefits in Japan is much narrower than in other OECD countries.[22]

One of the reasons for this low percentage of disability benefit recipients in Japan is related to the classification system of disability in Japan (Katsumata 2008; Momose 2010). In Sweden and the United States, the disability benefits are based on the determination of earning capacity. On the other hand, the benefits are based on the determination of functional disability in Japan; the degree to which daily living capacity is limited. Yet this determination does not take the earning capacity into account. As a result, the "Survey on the Actual Living Conditions of People with Disabilities" conducted in 2005 and 2006 shows that about half of those who had no income did not receive any disability pensions (Momose 2010, 175).[23] These people have no choice other than to rely on their families.

In addition, Japanese expenditure on disability benefits relative to its GDP is deficient. Figure 3.10 shows the public expenditure (cash benefits only) on disability (including illness) in OECD countries in FY 2017 (OECD 2022). On average, 1.6% of GDP was spent as cash benefits for disability in

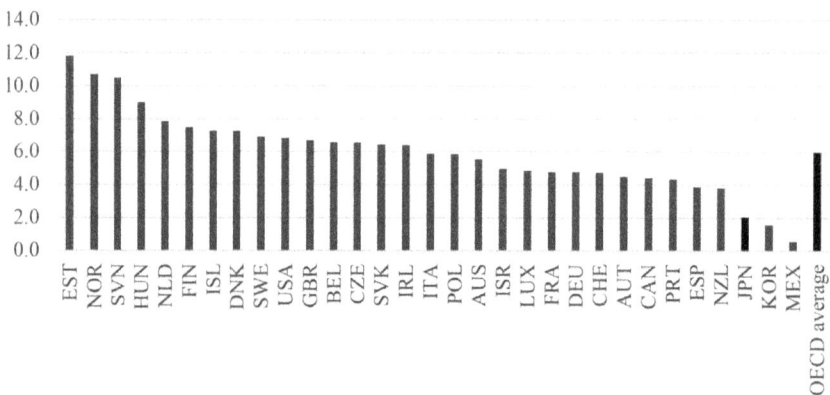

Figure 3.9   The Share of Disability Benefit Recipients in OECD Countries in %. *Source*: Created by the author based on data of OECD 2016 ("Figure 1.12. The share of disability benefit recipients is among the highest in OECD countries").http://dx.doi.org/10.1787 /888933323821.

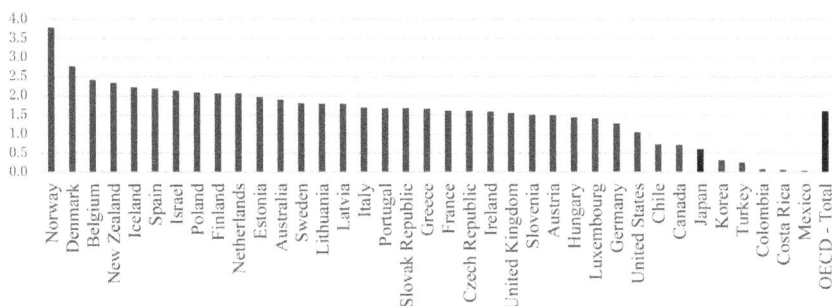

Figure 3.10   Public Expenditure on Disability and Sickness Cash Benefits in % of GDP. *Source*: Created by the author based on data from OECD "Social Expenditure—Aggregated data: Public expenditure on disability and sickness cash benefits, in % GDP" https://stats.oecd.org/Index.aspx?QueryId=33415.

OECD countries, but it was only about 0.6%, less than half of the average, in Japan. Only five countries (South Korea, Turkey, Colombia, Costa Rica, and Mexico) have a lower ratio than Japan.

Japan has a smaller range of de-commodification functions for the working-age population and a lower level of pension for the people with disability pensions than in other OECD countries. As a result, the range of people officially classified as "disabled" is limited, and even after the classification, the level of de-commodification by the disability benefits is far from sufficient. This narrow and limited disability pension makes the pension recipients dependent on their parents. The hikikomori problem for family also includes those disabled people living with their family (Sekimizu 2021).

Public Spending on Education

Historian of education Shinya Hashimoto points out that education provision can be considered a public benefit of the welfare state (Hashimoto 2013, 21–22). However, education provision is a unique benefit that functions as an accelerator of people's employability in the labor market (Hirota 2013, 244–245). Public spending on education aims to guarantee people's life security through the labor market by improving employability of people.

Kagawa, Kodama, and Aizawa (2014, 9) observe "In Japan, education up to high school is now considered as the de facto national minimum." High school graduation began to be expected as a standard educational achievement during the period of high economic growth. The high school enrollment rate varied from 35% to 70% depending on the prefecture in 1958, but it reached the 90% level in all prefectures in the 1980s (Kagawa, Kodama, and Aizawa 2014, 29) (cf. figure 3.11).[24]

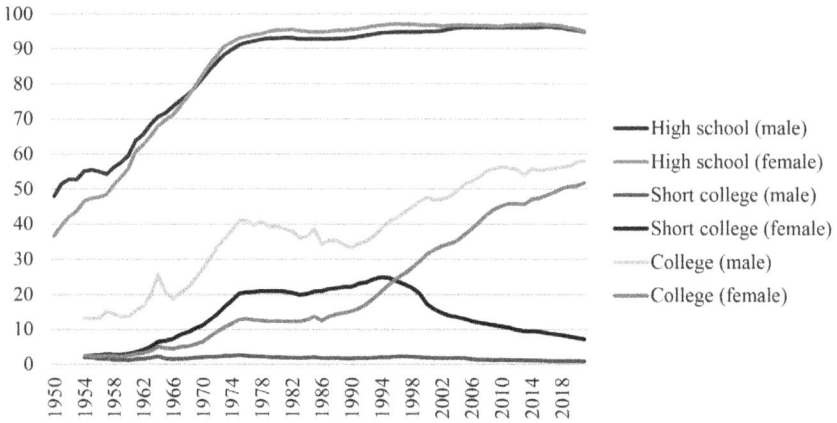

Figure 3.11   School Enrollment Rate. *Source*: Created by the author based on data from School Basic Survey.https://www.e-stat.go.jp/stat-search/files?page=1&layout=datalist &toukei=00400001&tstat=000001011528&cycle=0&tclass1=000001021812.

When most people go to high school, high school education comes to be seen as a prerequisite for getting a job. Sociologist of education Takehiko Kariya quotes farmers' words about their children's education from a study of the career paths of new graduates in Chiba Prefecture in the early 1960s. The following is a statement from a housewife from a medium-sized farm:

> We are sending our two children to high school, but our family is struggling to make ends meet. . . . Whether it's farming or getting a job, something has become difficult, and we need to give [our children] education. Those who go out to work (second and third sons and daughters) will not be able to become anything, and an heir who stays a farmer will feel inferior and not be able to talk to others in the village if they do not finish high school. It is common sense to educate them at high school. (Kariya 1995, 135)

He also quotes another poor farmer, who works at a candy factory: "High school is a normal education for people from now on. If the family budget permits, I want to send all my (six) children to high school. . . . It's a normal education, so if I make it that far, they'll be okay. They will be able to get out of this life" (Kariya 1995, 135–136).

Nowadays high school education does not give an advantage as an educational achievement in the labor market. In the 1960s, when the high school education rate expanded rapidly, the significance of a high school education shifted from "going to high school is an advantage" to "not going to high school is a disadvantage" (Kagawa, Kodama, and Aizawa 2014, 53–54).

Child psychiatrist Kazuhiro Takikawa, who is well known for his research on school non-attendance (*Futōkō*), pointed out that, since the 1970s, while competition for higher education has intensified, it has become difficult to find a positive meaning to go to school other than getting an education and getting a better job. This situation has led to an increase in school non-attendance (Takigawa 2012). Kazuki Ueyama (born in 1968) and Minoru Katsuyama (born in 1971), both mentioned in chapter 1, also pointed out their suffering resulting from attending competitive schools and studying hard just to get an education and to get a better job.

As the unemployment rate and the non-regular employment rate among youth have increased since the 1990s (figure 3.5), a higher education degree has become essential to compete in the labor market. However, the opportunity depends on the economic situation of the household of origin, because of the high proportion of private expenses necessary to receive higher education, and scholarships tend to be loans rather than benefits.[25]

LIFE SECURITY THROUGH THE FAMILY: PRE-COMMODIFICATION

The Historical Changes of the Family Role in Life Security

As already described, the role of the Japanese family for life security has been of great importance. Family sociologist Kizaemon Aruga explains its character and changes (Aruga [1965] 2001). This section mainly discusses Aruga's explanation of the role of the Japanese family for life security and its transformation.

According to Aruga, the modern Western family is "directly based on the humanism and individualism that emerged from the Christian tradition and supported by the enormous capitalism that developed along with it." To put it more concretely, under the conditions of capitalist development, "abundant external employments provided many opportunities for guaranteed life security, and parental responsibility for the support of children and their post-independence living was quickly released, making it easier for married couples to create families of one generation only" (Aruga [1965] 2001, 143–143).

On the other hand, the Japanese family system "had to secure the living of its members by managing the family business and family property for generations" and "the person who was responsible for managing the family system had to connect generations of the family system" (Aruga [1965] 2001, 143). In other words, the Japanese family system "had to have the character of an extremely self-protective group" which "took full responsibility for the life security of its members," and "the family members felt it their greatest duty to serve the longevity of the family system" (Aruga [1965] 2001, 145).

After World War II, the Japanese family system was regarded as "one of the roots of feudalism in Japan" and was strongly criticized. The family law was amended in 1947 to abolish the family system legally, but at the same time, "no new system, which guaranteed people's lives instead of the family system, was created in the chaotic society immediately after the defeat [of WWII]" (Aruga [1965] 2001, 149). Therefore, people had no choice but to keep relying on the family life security system.

With the "rapid development of industry and the resulting increase in employment" during high economic growth from the 1950s, "the responsibility of parents in the family system became less critical because the economic independence of children became much easier than before." This change occurred because "parents do not have to worry about the property of their branch of the family system, and the corporations where the children are employed can take over most of the responsibility for their life security" (Aruga [1965] 2001, 150).

Near the end of this article, Aruga describes the family's life security provision as follows: "The new nuclear family and the changed family system still have to be the last bastion of life security for its members, under the current situation where the economy is not yet large enough, the ideal of the welfare state has not yet been realized, and the conditions for social security are still too meager" (Aruga [1965] 2001, 152).

More than half a century has passed since Aruga wrote those words. Japan's economy has grown in size, and its GDP is now the third largest in the world. However, as we have already seen concerning the life security provided by the labor market and the government, Japanese society has not achieved "the ideal of the welfare state." As a result, the postwar nuclear family is yet to give up its responsibility for the life security of its members; Aruga's words are still true today: the nuclear family remains "the last bastion."

In addition to Aruga's explanation, the change in industrial structure, from a primary industry carried by self-employed and family workers to the secondary and tertiary industries with mainly employed workers, has been accompanied by an increase in nuclear families, modeled on the male-breadwinner and full-time housewife. This is because the nuclear family, which is also disembedded from the community, is a form of family that is compatible with the labor market. As section "Decline of Life Security through the Labor Market" considered, the role of life security for nuclear families has to increase as "the last bastion of life security for its members" when the exclusivity of the labor market increases with higher unemployment and more non-regular employment, and when the social security system is still underdeveloped.

Parental Duty to Support Immature Children

Although the revision of the family law after World War II abolished the intergenerational inheritance of the patriarchal family system legally, the duty of the family to provide life security has remained in the postwar Civil Code. The Civil Code, Article 877 paragraph 1, stipulates that "Lineal relatives by blood and siblings have a duty to support each other."[26] According to the prevailing interpretation of the family law, the nuclear family consisting of a married couple and their immature children is a *normative commune*. This normative commune holds the obligation of support as "a duty that should be shared down to the last remaining piece of meat" (Fukaya 1985, 203; Kojima 2016, 129).[27] In contrast, toward other relatives there is a duty to provide support only to the extent that it does not degrade their own standard of living.

The introduction of social security systems for elderly people has gradually reduced the duty of adult children to support their parents (Yamamoto 2009). These social security systems include: the National Health Insurance (1961), the National Pension Plan (1963), and the Long-Term Care Insurance (2000).

However, this is not the case with the parental responsibility to support their "immature" adult children. The duty of supporting children is said to continue until they reach "maturity." Maturity is considered a different standard than adulthood. While the distinction between adults and minors is age, the criterion for distinguishing between the mature and the immature is not age, but rather the person's "capacity for self-support for social survival" (cf. Higuchi 1988, 204–207). Jurist Norio Higuchi states as follows: "Although the content of the obligation changes as the child grows, the legal duty to provide support does not disappear completely. In other words, it may be said that the law on duty to support children recognizes or even reinforces the idea that parents will always be parents and children will always be children" (Higuchi 1988, 204).

A person can be regarded as immature even after reaching adulthood, in which case the parents still have an obligation to maintain his or her life security.[28] This indefinite duty of parents to support their immature children drives parents to urge their children to be independent of them.

Although there is almost no study on the case of hikikomori from the family law perspective, there is little doubt that the "immature child" interpretation is the key to interpreting the parental duty to support.[29] A civil law scholar, Matsuo Fukaya, argues that the key to understanding the immature child lies in the fact that the child is "growing toward maturity." In the case of "severe mental or physical disability" or "chronic illness," these issues are "of a different nature from the duty to maintain the life of an immature child" (Fukaya 1985, 227). However, as Fukaya admits, "the denotation of the immature child is not necessarily fixed." (Fukaya 1985, 228). The family law debates on how to interpret the immature child and the parental duty of supporting them, and the relationship between public and private support regarding this issue, have not reached a clear conclusion (Fukaya 1985, 228).[30]

When the life security provided by the welfare state is weak, and when children cannot receive life security from private corporations, the family inevitably continues to be expected to play the role, as Aruga put it, of "the last bastion of life security." So the hikikomori problem for family as a life security problem also has this legal context.

Non-intervention in the Family: The Case of School Non-attendance

As the Japanese social system still gives the family a significant obligation of life security of family members as the "last bastion of life security," the family unit is considered to have a great deal of discretion over the lives of its members. Hence the government is reluctant to intervene in the family unit in various cases, like child abuse, neglect, and domestic violence. This reluctance is the reverse side of the imposed responsibility of the family.

The approach to school non-attendance (*Futōkō*) is a clear example of the reluctance to intervene that is closely related to the hikikomori problem. According to Saitō and colleagues, "In the United States, children are not allowed to be absent without notification from their parents," and, in addition to that, "a doctor's note is usually required for prolonged absences (more than two weeks)" (Saitō et al. 2003, 1438–1439). If parents continue to keep the child at home, the school or other professionals (for example, psychiatrists or psychotherapists) will report the family to the police. Saitō observes:

> In the U.S., schools do not keep the [child's] problematic behavior in-house despite problem persistence. Failure to refer the child to a professional despite prolonged school refusal may be considered child neglect by the parents and the school, and legal action may be taken against the parents and the school. Some parents have children who have refused schooling since they lived in Japan and do not make active attempts to urge them to go to school even after moving to the U.S., as they did in Japan. Those parents are considered to be neglecting their children, and the school will suggest that the matter be reported to the police, and in some cases, schools actually have done so. (Saitō et al. 2003, 1439)

In the United States, parents cannot keep their children from going to school for an extended period. However, it is allowed in Japan. In Japan, the treatment of school refusal is considered a private family matter rather than a social matter that must involve professionals. This non-intervention, in turn, reinforces the responsibility of the family unit.

As a result, the inside of the family unit tends to be a black box, and it is difficult for people even to see whether the human rights of individuals are being protected within it. This black-box character of the Japanese family unit is also where so-called "strong family ties" are to be nurtured, yet at the same time, it can be a hotbed of various family-related problems. So the hikikomori problem as a life security problem for the family unit also ought to be situated within this context.

CONSIDERATIONS: THE HIKIKOMORI PROBLEM ROOTED IN POSTWAR JAPANESE SOCIETY

Familialistic Welfare Regime as a Social Foundation of the Hikikomori Problem

This chapter has examined the changes in life security roles in the private corporate sector, public sector, and the family unit. This section reflects on the arguments and clarifies the social structural context of the hikikomori problem. Figure 3.12 summarizes the discussion in previous sections.

In prewar Japanese society, the intergenerational succession of the family business and property was essential to secure the sustainability of family life security. The self-employed worker and family worker ratio was high: 69.3%

(1) Parents' indefinite obligation to provide life security measures for their immature children as a "last bastion of life security" even after the patriarchal extended family changed to nuclear family. (2) The public sector is reluctant to intervene in families as the other side of the coin of family responsibility.	(1) Provision of life security by private corporations to family units through male regular employees. (2) Since the late 1990s, the corporate welfare covers less employees due to increasing unemployment and non-regular employment. The corporate welfare for regular employees has also reduced.	(1) Underdeveloped welfare state relying on private sectors (corporate and family welfare). The small scale of disability benefits compared to OECD average. (2) The social security system consists of social insurance and public assistance and lacks social allowances (e.g., housing and family benefits).
		Life security by government
	Life security by labour market	
Life security by family		

Figure 3.12 **Division of Roles in Life Security Provision between Family, Market, and Government.** *Source*: Created by the author.

in 1920, 67.6% in 1930, and 58.0% even in 1940, when military industrialization was in full swing (Nomura 2014, 212). Most of the self-employed
were engaged in business to "earn income to support their families" (Nomura
2014, 236).

The commodification of labor power expanded drastically during the
period of rapid economic growth. The male-breadwinner model, which
distributes living wage to families through full-time male employees, was
the normative model of life security in Japan. The slowdown of economic
growth started in the 1970s. The government, which mainly focused on life
security via economic growth and pensions for older people who retired,
did not prepare a full-fledged welfare state in response to the economic
transformation, instead emphasizing the welfare society based on the family
and corporate welfare after the late 1970s, under the name of "the Japanese-
style of the welfare society."

Since the 1990s, non-regular employment has been growing and regular
employment shrinking, especially among the younger generation, so the
number of young people covered by the private corporate sector's life
security is decreasing. This shrinkage of corporate welfare has led inevitably
to an increased burden on family life security under the social policy of the
Japanese style of the welfare society.

In particular, families that do not have enough financial and emotional
security tend to experience difficulty supporting their children to get a job and
be included in corporate welfare. From the data on the users of the Community
Youth Support Center (*Chiiki Wakamono Sapōto Stēshon*),[31] it is possible to
estimate the types of youth struggling to find work. Michiko Miyamoto
(2015a) indicates that 40% of the Support Center users have experienced
school non-attendance (*Futōkō*), while approximately 25% have been bullied
at school. Dropout from high school, college, or university are 19.7%, and
35.6% have a high-school education or less as their final education.[32] In
addition, 26.4% have experienced financial difficulties at home, and 21.8%
have a family member receiving public assistance. More than 40% have
negative family backgrounds, such as child abuse, parents' separation and
bereavement, or a family member's mental illness. A total of 30% to almost
50% of the users have a diagnosis or suspicion of developmental disability
or mental illness.

To the questions this chapter posed—"why families are unable to find
other life security entities for their adult hikikomori children?" and "why
the jobless adult children continue to be excluded from the labor market,
public assistance, and other forms of life security and keep relying on their
families?"—the answer seems clear. In the familialism society, which lacks
public policy for the working population and imposes legal parental duty to
"immature" adult children, the family bears the responsibility of providing

care for their hikikomori children, especially under the condition of a shrinking labor market where people tend to be excluded from corporate welfare. The absence of public support for the working population also forces people who could not get included in the corporate welfare system to keep relying on their nuclear families.[33]

In this sense, the family cannot help but exert a kind of gravitational force that keeps family members in the parental household. In other words, the constellation of family life security, private corporate welfare, and the welfare state sets up a situation in which it is difficult for family members to leave the family. For the family, hikikomori cases do not necessarily mean those who never leave their room or home. It seems inexplicable that children who are spatially out of the house—who may be middle-aged or older—continue to be called "withdrawn" (*hikikomori*) children. However, it is easier to understand if we consider the following: use of the word "hikikomori" by the family is more about the gravitation itself than the behavior or condition of their children. The core of the hikikomori problem is this gravitation Japanese society has, which pushes away the "immature" citizen, who has difficulty becoming "independent," from social relationships and restricts them to their family household.

The Hikikomori Problem in the Modernization of Japanese Society

The construction of a full-fledged welfare state began in the early 1970s. However, the government soon abandoned that plan, and instead it introduced the policy of the Japanese style of the welfare society that emphasized corporate and family welfare in the late 1970s.[34] Family sociologist Emiko Ochiai points out that postwar Japanese society established a modern family system based on the "male-breadwinner" model, supplemented by a weak welfare state, and has been trying to maintain it. This combination of an underdeveloped welfare state and the modern family isolated from regional and kinship networks results in the "current situation in which the family is overburdened with insufficient socialization and marketization of care" (Ochiai 2013, 196–197).[35]

This modern Japanese social system has created the social structural context of the hikikomori problem for the family. The government has continued to prioritize the economy and kept social security for the working population as small as possible. The life security provided by the family assumes inclusion in corporate welfare as soon as the children graduate from school. However, because corporate welfare has shrunk since the 1990s, the modern Japanese nuclear family with jobless or precariously employed children confronts the problem of sustainability of family life security.

Many of those who drop out of the school-to-work transition system and enter the shelter of family life security often take a temporary break and then resume social activities such as job-seeking. In fact, the Cabinet Office surveys, which mainly define hikikomori as a state in which a person usually stays at home for six months or more, analyze the duration of withdrawal for those who have been hikikomori in the past. The results show that 70% of those in the 15–39 age group who experienced hikikomori in the past recovered from their hikikomori status within three years, and the majority of those in the 40–64 age group also lost it within three years (Cabinet Office 2016, 2019a).

As the survey of the Community Youth Support Center (Miyamoto 2015a) suggested, families that do not have enough financial and emotional security tend to have trouble supporting their children to get jobs and to be included in corporate welfare. The socioeconomic characteristics of the family have a significant impact on the occurrence of the hikikomori problem and on how they can deal with the problem.

However, this does not mean that the hikikomori problem does not occur in families with higher socioeconomic status. The hikikomori problem is rooted in the structural family responsibility for life security, including all aspects of their children. The fact that parents have socioeconomic resources does not necessarily mean that they can function as supports for their children. There are countless possibilities in which parental support for their children does not function well. Thus, while social stratification does exist, the hikikomori problem can arise in various forms in families of any class.

Toward the Comparative Study of Hikikomori Problems in Other Countries

The social conditions for the hikikomori problem for the family can be summarized as follows: (1) the modern nuclear family relies on the private corporate sector due to industrialization since the 1950s; (2) social security is underdeveloped due to the government's commitment to the economic-development-fast policy; and (3) the decline of the inclusive labor market severely affects disadvantaged families regarding, for example, financial capacity, educational achievement, and extra strength to support their children mentally.

Countries other than Japan would experience isolation cases in family units if they have the set of the following conditions: (1) the modern nuclear family is adapted to industrialization, (2) an underdeveloped social security system forces upon the nuclear family an infinite duty to care for their dependent members, and (3) there is a decline of an inclusive labor market. In a society where the nuclear family has the maximum responsibility for life security of its members, once the private corporate sector cannot absorb a certain number of people, the family has no choice but to hold them and take charge of their life security.

The problem of hikikomori for families has also arisen in European countries where a familialistic welfare regime is prominent. For example, southern European countries (Italy, Spain, and Portugal) were late to industrialize and are prominent in providing low direct subsidies to families (Esping-Andersen 1999, 60–63).[36] According to psychiatrist Tamaki Saitō, "Italy is the country where hikikomori became a social problem the earliest among EU countries" (Saitō 2015, 1569). In Spain, the term hikikomori has recently gained attention, and several studies have been published and argue the need for outreach to intervene with families (Ovejero et al. 2014; Malagón-Amor et al. 2015).[37]

Tamaki Saitō interprets this family welfare in the form of pre-commodification by linking it to Confucian culture and parents-children cohabitation culture (Saitō [2003] 2016, 124–126). He argues that the Confucian idea of "staying at home and taking care of parents is a desirable form of maturity" is linked to the acceptance of hikikomori cases.

However, I argue that many aspects of "Confucian culture" should be reinterpreted as a social system of a familialistic welfare regime. There are three reasons for this. First, the cultural factors of people's awareness or mindset are not the only factors that cause the problem of hikikomori for the family. Welfare sociologist Yasuhiro Kamimura has made the following points regarding elderly-parent support in South Korea. In South Korea, only a few percent of the elderly believe that their children should take care of the living expenses of their aged parents, but in reality 50% of the elderly are supported by their children. Even though the family support norm has become an old-fashioned concept, the inadequacy of the public pension system continues to require children to support their elderly parents (Kamimura 2015, 68–70). In the same way, even if the family is consciously detached from the family norm of supporting a hikikomori adult child, the family would have no choice but to take on the obligation to provide the life security of the "immature" adult child by the stipulates of a family law and the absence of public support system.

Second, the concept of Confucian culture can encompass various aspects of the family norm, so it is too wide and somewhat confusing when considering the hikikomori problem for the family. It is necessary to articulate the concept of Confucian culture in more concrete aspects of family life security. Family life security would cover almost all aspects of life, including financial support, housing, care provision, and food provision, and this is especially true in familialistic countries where the family holds the indefinite responsibility for the family unit. By thinking of the hikikomori problem for the family from the welfare regime perspective, we could think about how the welfare state can substitute for or support the family life security functions with, for example, housing allowances, disability pensions, basic income support.

Third, a Confucian culture perspective also prevents us from considering the social stratification background of families with hikikomori people, yet there are surveys that point to the socioeconomic background of the hikikomori problem as a family issue.

CONCLUSION

This chapter argued that the core of the hikikomori problem for families is anxiety over the life security of the family unit and examined why the family must experience the hikikomori problem as a life security problem. Parents hold the indefinite and permanent obligation to take care of their children unless private corporate welfare includes them. Therefore, it seems inevitable for parents to put severe pressures on their hikikomori children to get jobs as soon as possible in such an institutional condition. However, as I discussed, the question of "why don't you work?" drives hikikomori subjects into a corner and creates a vicious circle (see chapter 1).

The modern family is not so strong that it can sustain the indefinite life security of its members. Moreover, the instability of the family has increased due to the deteriorating employment environment and the increasing divorce rate in recent years. Countries such as Japan, Italy, and Spain—which have a solid familialistic character with less public support for families—also have low fertility rates (Esping-Andersen 2001, 80). There is an apparent limitation to burdening the family with indefinite life security functions. The hikikomori problem for the Japanese family can be interpreted as a cry against the overburdened obligations on them.

The hikikomori problem raises considerations over the redistribution of responsibility for life security. Of course, the division of roles in life security is not a matter of choice between the government, the market, and the family—but how to construct collaborative relationships among them and other factors like local community still needs to be addressed. As the next chapter will discuss, a new policy line has emerged since the 2000s that aims to shift the responsibility of life security measures to the local community (in addition to private corporations and families). There is enormous expectation that community welfare measures will support hikikomori cases. However, this policy line seems to actively avoid the increased governmental responsibility of life security provisions for jobless adults, as if it is just an evolved form of the older Japanese style of welfare society policy.

We also should not ignore the hikikomori subjects' perspective. The support they need is not identical with that of the family. We will return to the hikikomori experience in chapter 5.

NOTES

1. This association was established in Saitama Prefecture in 1999 as the "Hikikomori KHJ Parents Association" (*Hikikomori KHJ Oya no Kai*). In 2000, the name was changed to "National Association of Hikikomori KHJ Parents Associations" [*Zenkoku Hikikomori KHJ Oya no Kai (Kazokukai Rengōkai)*], and in 2004 it was incorporated as a nonprofit organization (Nagatomi and Moriguchi 2005, 14). Since its establishment, this group has been actively lobbying the Ministry of Health, Labor and Welfare and members of the Diet and politicians, requesting the government to take action regarding the hikikomori problem. In 2015, a new constitution of the group was established, and the official name was changed to "KHJ National Federation of Families with Hikikomori" (*KHJ Zenkoku Hikikomori Kazokukai Rengōkai*). KHJ originally was an abbreviation for Obsessive Compulsive Nervous Disorder (*Kyōhakusei Shinkei Shōgai*), Paranoia (*Higai Mōsō*), Personality Disorder (*Jinkaku Shōgai*), but it is officially an abbreviation for Family (*Kazoku*), *Hikikomori*, *Japan* in the new constitution of the association since 2015.

2. The total number of responses was 383. The relationship of the respondent to a hikikomori case was as follows: 62.9% were mothers, 31.1% fathers, 1.0% others, and 5.0% unknown (KHJ 2010). Thus, most of the respondents were parents of hikikomori children.

3. According to the research design in the report, this survey mainly targeted "families with ex-hikikomori people" (Tokyo Metropolitan Youth and Public Safety Headquarters 2009, 9). However, the responses from this survey regarding "the frequency of going out" show that 6% go out "every day for work or school," 6% go out "3–4 days a week for work or school," 2% go out "frequently for fun, and so on (e.g., funerals and weddings)," 5% go out "occasionally to socialize," 38% go out "only for their hobbies," 25% go out "to the convenience store," 13% go out "from their room but never leave the house": and 2% "never leave their room": and 3 % give "No Answer." The sum of those who don't leave home is 15%. Although this survey says the main target of the family survey is families with ex-hikikomori people, there is not much difference compared to the KHJ surveys aforementioned. Regarding the basic information of the respondents, 74% of the respondents were mothers, and 20% were fathers (Tokyo Metropolitan Youth and Public Safety Headquarters 2009, 67). As for the age distribution of the respondents' children, 8.1% were under 19 years old, 19.5% in their early 20s, 22.7% in their late 20s, 22.6% in their early 30s, 22.6% in their late 30s, and 5.4% in their early 40s (Tokyo Metropolitan Youth and Public Safety Headquarters 2009, 69). There is also no significant difference with the age distribution in the KHJ surveys. Thus, this chapter refers to this survey data to identify the core of the hikikomori problem for families. For detailed information on how the

survey was conducted, see the Tokyo Metropolitan Youth and Public Safety Task Force (2009, 66–67).

4. The original figure is rearranged in order of the sum of the percentages of "Strongly agree" and "agree."

5. Regarding the gender and age of the hikikomori children, majority are male, and the average age is in their 30s. In the KHJ 2010 report, 76.0% were male, 19.7 % female, and 4.2% unidentified. The youngest case was 11 years old, the oldest was 55 years old, and the average age was 30.3 years (KHJ 2010). In the KHJ 2016 survey report, the percentage of males was 80.2%, and women was 16.8%. The average age was 34.1, the youngest was 14, the oldest was 53 (KHJ 2016).

6. Andy Furlong lists the following trends as factors in the increase of hikikomori youth in Japan: the government's lack of support for youth and neglect of the governmental responsibility for family care, as well as the Confucian concept of life-long reciprocal dependency in Japanese families, a monolithic and competitive education system, and changes in the labor market (the proportion of part-time employment and increased unemployment) among younger generations. This chapter shares his perspective by considering the broader social systems. However, I will not investigate the causes of the substantial increase in hikikomori, but rather ask the question why the hikikomori problem for families is considered a life security problem, and try to answer the question by applying welfare regime theory. This chapter will also complement Furlong's research by clarifying the structure of life security systems, which Furlong (2008) does not discuss. Akihiko Higuchi also provides the important insight that hikikomori is an "illusion" projected on the wall of "non-receipt of social services" (Higuchi 2008). This chapter will also develop Higuchi's suggestion by examining the tripartite relationship between the labor market, the government, and the family.

7. Ōsawa's discussion of "life security governance" is a model which reinterprets Esping-Andersen's welfare regimes from a gender perspective. She proposes the "male-breadwinner" type, the "balanced-support" type, and the "market-oriented" type as the three types of life security systems (Ōsawa 2013, 121–134). Political scientist Tarō Miyamoto also uses the term "life security" (Seikatsu Hoshō), which refers to "a system that makes people's lives sustainable." Its focus is on the "coordination of education, employment, and social security" (Miyamoto 2013, 1).

8. Esping-Andersen uses the term "state" in the explanation of the welfare regime, but I use the term "government" to avoid the wider meaning of the term "state," which can include the people of the nation state.

9. Social policy scholar Takafumi Uzuhashi lists ten items in the Japanese social security system: (1) unemployment insurance, (2) unemployment assistance, (3) public assistance, (4) benefits for the young unemployed, (5) housing benefits, (6) family benefits, (7) single-parent benefits, (8) employment conditional benefits, (9) income tax, and (10) legal minimum wage (Uzuhashi 2011, 134–135). These characteristics of the Japanese social security system will be discussed in "Life Security through the Government" of this chapter.

10. A total of 70–80% of the self-employed worker has been male, while 70–80% of family worker has been female.

11. Source: Labour Force Survey, Ministry of Internal Affairs and Communications. These figures are not particularly high among advanced capitalist countries. According to Nomura, "As of 2010, the ratio of self-employed workers to total workers was 11.6% in Germany and 7.0% in the U.S., while in Japan the ratio was 12.3%, almost the same. Japan has become, so to speak, a normal developed country" (Nomura 2014, 213–213).

12. The term "corporate welfare" in this chapter refers to the entire corporate provision for the life security of employees, including the living wage.

13. Keiichirō Hamaguchi says that it was the government that required companies to provide life security during World War II. "The wartime government-controlled labor mobility by prohibiting all hiring, job changes, and dismissals without governmental permission. It imposed three years training of skilled employees on medium-sized and larger companies. . . . The government also enforced an age-based wage system, 'focusing on securing a living for workers,' and instructed companies to introduce a monthly wage system for workers who had previously been paid on a daily basis. Industrial Patriots [*Sangyō Hōkokukai*] as labor-management consultative bodies were set up in companies across the country to support this." These policies were based on the "idea of treating the corporations as if they were branches of the state," and they intended to realize the "enforcement of life security on the companies" (Hamaguchi 2013b, 4).

14. According to Tachibanaki, corporate welfare such as retirement benefits and corporate pensions preceded public social security systems in not only Japan but also Europe and the United States (Tachibanaki 2005, Chap. 1). Companies enhanced corporate welfare in order to increase employee retention and productivity (Tachibanaki 2005, 87). In both Europe and Japan, large corporations initially began to provide family allowances, but in Europe they were gradually legislated as a social security system. In Japan, on the contrary, many employees thought that family allowances should be paid by private companies, and child allowances were not expanded as a social security system (Hamaguchi 2009, 128–130).

15. On the other hand, labor sociologist Kimiko Kimoto points out as follows: "The government developed public enterprises, public subsidies, and various industry protections to compensate for the low level of social security" for the "former middle class consisting of farmers and other self-employed workers" (Kimoto 2004, 305).

16. The minimum wage was socially accepted at a lower level than was needed to live on because, as non-regular employees were mainly housewives and students, they were positioned as "household supporting" labor on the premise that regular male employees (namely, husbands and fathers) earned living wages (Hamaguchi 2009, 113–118).

17. Source: The *Labour Force Survey* conducted by the Statistics Bureau of the Ministry of Internal Affairs and Communications.

18. Source: The *Labour Force Survey* conducted by the Statistics Bureau of the Ministry of Internal Affairs and Communications. Data are based on February data before 2001 and average data from January to March since 2002. Data for 15–24-year-old group exclude those who attend school and for the sake of clarity,

data for those aged 65 and over, who have a high rate of non-regular employment, have been excluded.

19. Source: Data provided by the Japan Institute for Labour Policy and Training based on the Labour Force Survey by the Ministry of Internal Affairs and Communications.

20. The rates of households receiving housing allowances in each country are all figures for the first half of the 2000s. Public housing (social housing) provision is also small in Japan. The percentage of public housing among the whole rental housing provision is 6.1% in Japan, compared to 17% in France, 35% in the Netherlands, and 17% in Sweden (Hirayama 2011, 12, 17). Urban policy scholar Yoshihito Honma points out that Japan's housing policy has focused "only on measures to acquire owner-occupied houses, which are directly linked to economic stimulus," and has neglected the concept of "the right to housing as a human right" (Honma 2009, iii–v).

21. The following is the note to the figure in the OECD report (OECD 2016): "Disability benefits include benefits received from schemes to which beneficiaries have paid contributions (contributory), programs financed by general taxation (non-contributory) and work injury schemes. The last available year is 2014 for Estonia; 2013 for Australia, Czech Republic, Finland and the United States; 2010 for Spain; 2009 for Mexico; 2008 for Austria, Japan and Korea; 2007 for Canada and France; 2005 for Luxembourg."

22. The OECD paper presents an argument to "reduce . . . the generous sickness and disability benefit system" in Nordic countries (OECD 2016, 32). However, this chapter argues that it is these "generous benefits" that reduce the family responsibility to ensure the life security of immature children.

23. On the other hand, about 20% of those who earn 200,000 yen (approximately 1,800 US dollars) or more per month as an employed person receive a disability pension of 1 million yen (approximately 9,000 US dollars) or more per year (Momose 2010, 173).

24. Source: Ministry of Education, Culture, Sports, Science and Technology, Basic School Survey.

25. Although the Japanese public and private expenditure on education (4.95%) is not so different from the OECD average expenditure on education (5.33%), the characteristic of Japanese spending on education is the high ratio of private spending to total spending (OECD 2015, 226). Private spending on education is not particularly high below the secondary (high school) level in Japan. However, private spending for higher education accounts for about 65%. The only country which has a higher number than Japan is South Korea (OECD 2015, 238).

26. The English translations of laws are cited from the website of the Ministry of Justice, "Japanese Law Translation" (http://www.japaneselawtranslation.go.jp/).

27. This interpretation was first published by Zennosuke Nakagawa in 1928 in "The Essence of the Kinship Obligation to Support," and is still the prevailing theory and precedent today (Fukaya 1985, 203; Kojima 2016, 129).

28. Regarding the parental duty of support to an adult immature child, for example, there is a court case in which the Tokyo High Court ruled in 2010 on the "parental duty of support to an adult child who is still in college" (Hayano 2015; Kojima 2016,

136). This case is as follows. After the parents divorced, the father continued to pay child support to the separated child until the child reached adulthood, but the child sued for payment of tuition and living expenses while in college. The first trial court did not recognize the necessity of payment, but the second trial court reversed the first trial court's decision and approved the payment of part of the tuition and living expenses until the child graduated from college. In another case (concluded in 1976), the Tokyo High Court ruled that the father could be ordered to pay living expenses for a child living with the mother as an immature child, even if the child had reached the age of majority (Kojima 2016, 136).

29. Lawyer Atsushi Hirata mentions that academic discussion on the duty to support is not active and he offers two reasons for this. One is the Japanese law of duty to support is unique apart from the original foundation of Italian and French civil law. The other is the difficulty of the relationship between the Public Assistance Law and the duty of support in the Civil Code (Hirata 2020, 1).

30. Jurist Atsuko Miyake introduces the view that the parental duty to take care of immature children arises during the transitional period until the obligation of the welfare state has been established. However, Miyake herself concludes that both the parental duty and the public responsibility (such as child allowance) should be strengthened (Miyake 1999).

31. In 2006, the Ministry of Health, Labor, and Welfare launched this project in 25 locations nationwide as a public service to support young people who are failing to find work. See chapter 4.

32. The detailed numbers are as follows: 6.3% have a junior high school education, 7.9% have dropped out of high school, and 21.4% have a high school education. Those who attended part-time or correspondence high schools were 21.0%, which is higher than the average for those of the same age (Miyamoto 2015a, 19).

33. Inui et al. examine the relationship between the youth difficulty to leave the parental house and the provision of public support in a comparison between Japanese and U.K. data. The analysis suggests the following: (1) Japanese youth find it difficult to get out of non-regular work; (2) Japanese male youth experience difficulty in leaving their parental house and forming a family when they have a non-regular job; and (3) U.K. youth have a high rate of social security recipients and the number is highest when they are leaving the parental house, but this correlation is not observed in Japanese youth (Inui et al. 2021).

34. Uzuhashi summarizes the characteristics of the late developed welfare state in the following four points (Uzuhashi 2011, 54–55). (1) While public welfare remains low, families and corporations substitute for the welfare function. (2) Rapid industrialization forces workers to make enormous sacrifices, and the state has to intervene in working hours and hygiene standards. (3) The state has characteristics of developmentalism, which places a high policy priority on creating and providing employment opportunities through economic growth, and welfare policies focus on self-independence through employment. (4) A "lagging effect" is obtained in which the level of social expenditure as a percentage of GDP remains low, but this effect is eventually lost. The "lagging effect" (lagging benefit) that Uzuhashi refers to here is due to the existence of a young population structure (i.e., a productive young labor

force), the provision of domestic care work by family members, and the existence of social norms that support family care. These characteristics exactly hold to the Japanese-style of the welfare society.

35. Political scientist Tarō Miyamoto characterizes the position of the Japanese welfare state as "the midpoint between the welfare models of the advanced industrialized countries and the later East Asian models" (Miyamoto 2013, 28).

36. See Uzuhashi (2011, 45–48) for a discussion of the classification of Southern European welfare states as latecomer welfare states.

37. Even in East Asian countries which rely on kinship networks for family care work, the problem of life security for families is expected to arise once the demographic bonus disappears (cf. Ochiai 2013, 197).

Chapter 4

Discourses on the Hikikomori Problem from the 1980s to the 2010s

WHAT IS THE HIKIKOMORI PROBLEM?

This chapter examines discourses of the government and other representative figures regarding the hikikomori problem between the 1980s and the 2010s and aims to clarify the framework for understanding the hikikomori problem and its transformation in those discourses during that period.

Ishikawa (2007), Takayama (2008), Kudō (2008), and Kudō (2013) have already attempted to analyze the discourse on the hikikomori problem. Ishikawa refers to the changes in the number of newspaper articles and the atmosphere in her research field from the late 1980s to the early 2000s (Ishikawa 2007, Chap. 2). Takayama (2008) analyzes the hikikomori discourse up to the 1990s concerning its connection with the discourse on school non-attendance (*Futōkō*) (Takayama 2008, 44). Kudō (2008) analyzes the hikikomori discourse from the 2000s onward. He finds that criminal cases in the early 2000s triggered the perception of the hikikomori problem as a "criminal risk" and a target of psychiatric treatment. Furthermore, the context of employment issues also emerged, and the discourse on hikikomori has fluctuated between the two contexts of psychiatric issues and employment issues. Kudō (2013) focuses on the Ministry of Health, Labour, and Welfare (MHLW)'s "Guideline for Community Mental Health Activities Regarding Social Withdrawal [*Shakaiteki Hikikomori*]," a provisional version of which was published in 2001. He argues that community mental health professionals tried to screen the hikikomori cases with decisive biological factors for which medication is adequate from the hikikomori cases without such biological factors.

While these previous studies aimed to clarify the discursive history and discursive formation of the hikikomori problem, this chapter focuses on the government's and proponents' framework for understanding the problem. To analyze the framework for understanding the problem is to clarify what condition they understood as hikikomori, how they understood its cause, and what measures they proposed to address the problem. Thus, this chapter focuses on the definition, the cause, and the treatment of the hikikomori in those discourses. The reason why it is important to treat the governmental and other proponents' discourses is to clarify the authority of the framework for understanding the hikikomori problem. In addition, these discourses influenced or articulated policies to address the hikikomori problem. Therefore, this chapter also examines some policies for the hikikomori problem, which were realized based on governmental and other proponents' discourse.

THE DISCOVERY AND EXTENT: FROM THE LATE 1980S TO THE LATE 1990S

The Late 1980s

This section examines representative discourses from the end of the 1980s to the late 1990s. In the late 1980s, several articles and policy documents started to address the hikikomori problem. Among only a few articles mentioning the term "hikikomori," three texts of the hikikomori problem are taken up here: (1) the article "Dropouts, Apathy, and Hikikomori" published in *Education and Medicine* in 1986, (2) *Children's Relationship Disorders* published in 1989, and (3) "Toward the Realization of Comprehensive Youth Measures" by the Council on Youth Affairs in 1989. The authors of two of the three articles were education scholars because the first focus on the hikikomori problem was in the context of education. Let us examine the framework for understanding the problem in these texts.

"Dropouts, Apathy, and Hikikomori" (May 1986)

One of the first articles to use the term "hikikomori" was "Dropouts [*Ochikobore*], Apathy, and Hikikomori," published in Volume 34, Number 5 of *Education and Medicine* (*Kyōiku to Igaku*) in May 1986. The author was Michihiko Kitao, a professor at Osaka Kyoiku University specializing in educational psychology.

Kitao wrote the following about hikikomori: "There are many cases where students drop out, become apathetic, and withdraw into their own shells. These cases must be emphasized as emotional disorders created by today's schools" (Kitao 1986, 38).[1] According to Kitao, the background to apathy is a lack of "real experience in the real world," which means "knowing little outside the world of school and study" (Kitao 1986, 39).

The school system, which requires homogeneous evaluation, creates these dropout children, and "the failure to conform to the group" injures these children—only a school system which acknowledges heterogeneity as individuality can provide a fundamental solution (Kitao 1986, 39). The cases discussed in this article are those of elementary school and junior high school students. While overlapping with the concept of school non-attendance, hikikomori focuses on the emotional aspect of helplessness and perceived inferiority of those dropped-out children.

Kitao argues that hikikomori is a problem of "school mental health" and positions it as a problem created by a school system that imposes uniform evaluation standards on children. Thus, his framework understands the hikikomori problem as a school system problem that educational administration must rectify.

Children's Relationship Disorders (October 1989)

Children's Relationship Disorders, published in October 1989, devoted a chapter to "social withdrawal [*Shakaiteki Hikikomori*]" along with other topics (e.g., selective silence, bullying, school refusal, and autism). The author was Masahiko Sugiyama, a PhD in education who worked on the rehabilitation of autistic children.

Sugiyama defined hikikomori as children who "for various reasons, . . . have difficulty in taking an active role in situations where they have to collaborate in social interaction and groups. This results in learning behaviors that avoid or minimize exposure to such situations" (Sugiyama 1989, 31). According to Sugiyama, hikikomori is a deviation from age-appropriate social interactions. He assumes that hikikomori connotes any condition in which a child is unable to engage in "appropriate social behavior" in the course of his/her development (Sugiyama 1989, 30) and "does not actively participate in or avoids social interaction or group activities" (Sugiyama 1989, 32). He takes up the cases of a three-year-old and a junior high school student. Considering the condition of a three-year-old child as "hikikomori" is not common in contemporary usage of the term. However, he expects such deviations from normal interactions even in three-year-old children.

Sugiyama understands hikikomori as a problem caused by individual disability and the parent-child relationship in the home environment. Thus, his framework assumes that parents and education professionals ought to be the primary problem solvers. He admits that "the causes and the process which form the hikikomori condition are diverse," but he lists the causes of hikikomori cases as the following: "failure of the home environment," "so-called 'overprotection [*Kahogo*],'" "excessive instruction or punishment [by parents]," and "a degree of disability."[2]

The Council on Youth Affairs, Opinion Report: "Toward the
Realization of Comprehensive Youth Measures" (June 1989)

In June 1989, the Council on Youth Affairs, an advisory body established
within the Ministry of Internal Affairs and Communications (*Seishōnen
Mondai Shingikai*), submitted a report to the prime minister titled "Toward
the Realization of Comprehensive Youth Measures," the introduction of
which stated that "an increase in asocial behavior" had emerged as a "youth
problem" in addition to the traditional "delinquency." Furthermore, chapter
1, titled "Location of the Problem and Perspectives for Consideration,"
mentions hikikomori as follows: "Recently, bullying and school violence
seem to be declining, but new problems such as hikikomori and school refusal
[*Tōkō Kyohi*], especially among adolescents, have arisen, and the situation is
alarming" (Council on Youth Affairs 1989, Chap. I).

The increase in hikikomori and school refusal is a "new problem," and the
background to these problems is the emergence of "affluent society" since the
late 1980s (Council on Youth Affairs 1989, section II-1). Why does affluent
society produce asocial behavior? The report explains: "Young people who
grow up among today's material wealth and convenience are beginning to
lack spiritual wealth [*Kokoro no Yutakasa*] and mental toughness [*seishinteki
na Takumashisa*]" (Council on Youth Affairs 1989, section II-1).

According to the report, material wealth undermines spiritual wealth and
mental toughness. It is not clear what is meant by "spiritual wealth" and
"mental toughness" here, but this report repeats that "material wealth" has
deprived youth of "spiritual wealth" and "mental toughness" as follows: "We
believe that it is crucial for those involved in developing youth to make more
tremendous efforts to restore the basic things that are often lost among youth
today in exchange for material wealth and convenience of living, i.e., spiritual
wealth and the ability to live toughly" (Council on Youth Affairs 1989, Chap.
I). This report requires more efforts of those involved in developing youth to
regain their spiritual wealth and mental toughness. "Those who support youth
development" include "private organizations and the government," which
cover "a wide range of fields, including education, welfare, labor, protection,
correction, and other fields related to youth development" (Council on Youth
Affairs 1989, section II-3).

How do these private and governmental organizations deal with
the hikikomori problem? The section "Dealing with so-called mental
maladjustment problems" discusses the treatment of hikikomori and school
non-attendance (*Futōkō*). It says: "a comprehensive counseling facility that
provides the functions of therapeutic measures, including psychotherapy and
medical treatment, and counseling and guidance measures" is necessary to
treat the "asocial behavior" of youth.

At the same time, however, the report also emphasizes the responsibility of the family to work on this asocial youth problem:

> There was a strong comment on the importance of the family as a place that should play a fundamental role in the human development of youth, the significance of cooperative and stable family life in preventing problematic behaviors, and especially the importance of the warm affection of parents during infancy and the discipline of the family during childhood. There was an opinion that these points should be further emphasized in the future. (Council on Youth Affairs 1989, Introduction)

The report notes the recognition that "it is not clear whether the youth face a problem or not at first glance" (Council on Youth Affairs 1989, section II-2) and emphasizes the responsibility of both the government and the family as the entities that deal with youth problems.

This report understands that the backgrounds of the asocial behavior of hikikomori are the economic and social changes in Japanese society that have achieved "material wealth" and convenience. It also suggests that families must provide affection and discipline to youth, and specialized organizations must be established to provide therapy and guidance for youth.

Summary of the Discourse in the Late 1980s

Education professionals started to discuss the hikikomori problem in the late 1980s. They suggested broad elements as causes of the problematic behavior, from individual to social structural factors: school systems that impose uniform evaluation standards, overprotective parent-child relationships, or disabilities of children. The first governmental discourse appeared at the end of the 1980s, and it focused on material wealth and convenience, which had deprived youth of mental toughness. It recommended psychotherapy and educational instruction as the measures to treat the problem and, at the same time, underlined responsibility of the family.

The Early 1990s

For the first half of the 1990s, this section focuses on (1) *White Paper on Youth: Current Situation and Measures for Youth Problems*, (2) *Report of the Council on Youth Affairs*, (3) *Departure from Hikikomori* by psychological counselor Fujiya Tomita, and (4) *Hikikomori Q&A* by psychiatrist Hiroshi Inamura.

White Paper on Youth: Current Situation and Measures for Youth Problems (January 1990)

The Youth Affairs Headquarters of the Ministry of Internal Affairs and Communications compiled and published the *White Paper on Youth: Current Situation and Measures for Youth Problems* (*Seishōnen Hakusho: Seishōnen Mondai no Genjō to Taisaku*) in January 1990, partly based on the Council on Youth Affairs opinion mentioned in the previous chapter. The white paper begins as follows:

> The sound development of the youth who will lead our country's next generation is a national challenge. Regarding the current state of youth problems, it has been pointed out that youth generally lack spiritual wealth and mental toughness amid progress in economic affluence and convenience of living. In addition, juvenile delinquency is still at a high level, mainly in the form of initial delinquency such as shoplifting, and in recent years, a new problem has arisen in the form of an increase in, e.g., hikikomori and school refusal. (Youth Affairs Headquarters 1990, 3)

In response to the opinions of the Council on Youth Affairs in the previous year, this white paper divided the problematic behavior of youth into *problematic antisocial behavior* and *problematic asocial behavior*. It took up hikikomori as an example of the latter, along with apathy, school refusal, and suicide (Youth Affairs Headquarters 1990, 27–28).

> In recent years, experts have pointed out that cases of hikikomori and apathy are on the rise. Although it is challenging to define them strictly, hikikomori refers to those who try to minimize contact with family members and people outside the family, for example, staying in one's room all day or taking meals alone in one's room. Apathy refers to, for example, those who lose interest in their academic or professional life and spend their days in idleness. In the case of college students, this is known as student apathy. (Youth Affairs Headquarters 1990, 27–28)

This paper positions problematic asocial behaviors in the context of the problem of "spiritual wealth" that arises after "economic wealth" has been achieved, but it does not specify who ought to be responsible for treating the problem. There is emphasis on neither "social independence" nor "employment," both of which the government has often emphasized since the 2000s.

Model Project for Welfare Measures for Hikikomori and School Non-Attendance Children (April 1991)

The Ministry of Health and Welfare (MHW) launched the "Model Project for Welfare Measures for Hikikomori and School Refusal Children" (*Hikikomori*

Futōkō Jidō Fukushi Taisaku Moderu Jigyō) in April 1991. This model project is based on the Child Welfare Law and is limited to those under 18. Therefore, the main target of this project is children who refuse to go to school; hikikomori youth more than 18 years old are excluded from this project.[3] According to Shiokura ([1999] 2001), the bureaucrat in charge of this project said the term "hikikomori" "is a word that expresses the 'state' of staying at home and not being able to go out. There is no technical definition" (Shiokura [1999] 2001, 24). It is difficult to determine the exact relationship between this MHW project and the Council on Youth Affairs opinion report in 1989, even upon examination of the minutes of the House of Representatives Committee on Education (February 20, 1999). However, this program provides the counseling and guidance function that the opinion report proposed.[4]

Report of the Council on Youth Affairs, Basic Measures to Deal with Youth Apathy, Hikikomori, and Other Problematic Behaviors: Toward the Development of Youth with Vitality (December 1991)

In response to the opinions expressed by the Council on Youth Affairs in June 1989, in December of that year Toshiki Kaifu, the prime minister at that time, instructed the Council on Youth Affairs to prepare a report on the issue, which was delivered in October 1991 and titled "Basic Measures to Deal with Youth Apathy, Hikikomori, and Other Problematic Behaviors: Toward the Development of Youth with Vitality" (Council on Youth Affairs 1991).

The report states: "Unlike antisocial problem behaviors such as delinquency, the recent surge in asocial problem behaviors such as apathy and hikikomori is a new situation that we have not seen before, and it is alarming" (Council on Youth Affairs 1991, 9).[5]

The latter half of the report presented measures to deal with this problem which superseded the policy put forward in the 1989 Opinion Report. It called for appropriate responses at home, school, in the community, and the workplace, and advocating the need for measures such as the enhancement and reinforcement of new counseling and guidance functions for youth that professionally deal with problematic asocial behaviors, and the enhancement of professional functions by psychiatrists and psychologists (Council on Youth Affairs 1991, 12–13).

Fujiya Tomita, Departure from Hikikomori: A Heartfelt Record of Children Who Refuse to Go to School, Refuse to Work, and Reject Human Beings (September 1992)

In 1990, Fujiya Tomita started supporting hikikomori children and established "Friend Space" as a free space outside the home in Matsudo, Chiba

Prefecture. Throughout the 1990s, Tomita frequently appeared in newspaper reports referring to the hikikomori problem. In 1992, he published a book about hikikomori titled *Departure from Hikikomori: A Heartfelt Record of Children Who Refuse to Go to School, Refuse to Work, and Reject Human Beings*. This book was the first one on the market with the word "hikikomori" in its title. Tomita wrote:

> It is only in the last five years or so that I have become aware of the word "hikikomori." I have been working with families for more than ten years, who suffer from the refusal of school and work, and recently I have been meeting more and more youth, including these children, who have been refusing to interact with others for a long time, as if they were rejecting human beings. I have also noticed an increase in those who show this tendency among junior high school students. Then, at the end of the year before last (the year 1990), I read an article that the Ministry of Health and Welfare negotiated with the Ministry of Finance for a budget for a "model project for welfare measures for hikikomori and school non-attendance children." This article made me aware that hikikomori had become a social problem. (Tomita 1992, 19)

According to Tomita, hikikomori is essentially a rejection of human beings, and "the problem is not whether they go to school or not, but whether they reject human relationships or not" (Tomita 1992, 207). Thus, even if children go to school, if they reject human relationships, they are hikikomori. However, on the other hand, even if they do not go to school, they are not hikikomori if they still engage in human relationships. The hikikomori is in an ambivalent state where he/she rejects relationships with others, even though he/she wants to have relationships with others.

Tomita disagrees with the view that hikikomori is an individual pathology, arguing that hikikomori is "one of a wide variety of socially pathological phenomena" (Tomita 1992, 151). He contends that hikikomori is "one of the phenomena created by modern society," and "it is necessary to understand the feelings of children who can barely maintain their existence by being hikikomori" (Tomita 1992, 41). He singles out two aspects of modern society that create the hikikomori phenomenon: (1) an overwhelming lack of opportunities to learn the basics of interpersonal relationships naturally, leading to a loss of the "basic construction of human relationships" (Tomita 1992, 31); and (2) "modern education that tries to fit [children] into the mold of uniform 'common sense' that adults believe in" (Tomita 1992, 40).

Although hikikomori is not a mental illness, and hikikomori is not subject to psychiatric treatment (Tomita 1992, 148), Tomita contends that hikikomori and mental illness are different but overlapping problems. Tomita says that there are cases where mental illness is the cause of hikikomori and vice versa. He says:

> In some cases, repressed school refusal or hikikomori may become "illness," while in other cases, school refusal or hikikomori may be caused by "illness." Obviously, some need medical care, and others do not, even among [the similar condition of] children who do not go to school or work. It seems challenging for conventional psychiatry to discern the difference, and even "experts" are struggling to "diagnose." (Tomita 1992, 150–151)

He does not deny that there are cases where hikikomori and mental illness overlap, such that medical treatment is necessary.

Tomita also acknowledges the rationalization by society and the school education system as contributing factors to the hikikomori problem. He suggests that support people should not regard hikikomori as mentally ill subjects of psychiatric treatment but rather "stay close" to the subjective experience of conflict.

Hiroshi Inamura, School Refusal and Hikikomori Q&A (September 1993)

In 1993, a year after the publication of *Departure from Hikikomori*, psychiatrist Hiroshi Inamura published *School Refusal and Hikikomori Q&A*. The book is written in a question-and-answer style; most of the questions are from mothers about their children's problems.

Although there is no clear definition of hikikomori in this book, Inamura describes it as "a kind of disorder in a broad sense, and if it is not dealt with appropriately, it will really become worse" (Inamura 1993, 84). Inamura also observes that "there are many cases of school refusal and hikikomori that are suspected to be psychosis" (Inamura 1993, 193). He frequently refers to hikikomori as a mental illness and calls for treatment by psychiatrists. Hikikomori is undoubtedly a subject of psychiatric treatment for Inamura, and he promoted medicalization of this problem, in sharp contrast to Tomita, who argues that hikikomori is neither a disorder nor an illness.

Summary of the Early 1990s

In the first half of the 1990s, arguments from proponents of different positions emerged; a major point of contention concerned the relationship between hikikomori and mental illness. Although Tomita and Inamura both consider hikikomori asocial behaviors that deviate from the normative social behavior, especially attending school and work, they were sharply different in terms of their involvement with psychiatry. Tomita argued that hikikomori is not a subject of psychiatric pathology but of a conflict over the refusal of human relations, although he did not deny the utility of psychiatric treatment. On the other hand, Inamura, a psychiatrist, emphasized the need for psychiatric treatment for hikikomori cases.

The Council on Youth Affairs first raised youth's asocial behavior in the 1989 report and even suggested the need for professional institutions to deal with it. The council called for enhancing therapeutic treatment and consultation and guidance by professionals for asocial behaviors. Therefore, it affirms those treatments, including psychiatry. At the same time, the MHL started a program for hikikomori children under 18 years old. However, administrative documents rarely mentioned hikikomori after this during the 1990s. As will be explained later, it was not until the 2000s that the government mentioned the hikikomori problem again.

The Late 1990s

This section examines three books: (1) Sadatsugu Kudō's *Hey, Hikikomori: It's Time to Go Outside*, (2) *Japanese Journal of Clinical Psychiatry*, which featured a special issue titled "Psychopathology of Hikikomori," and (3) Tamaki Saitō's *Shaikaiteki Hikikomori*.

Sadatsugu Kudō, Hey, Hikikomori: It's Time to Go Outside (August 1997)

Sadatsugu Kudō, who ran the private school "Tame-Juku," published *Hey, Hikikomori: It's Time to Go Outside* in August 1997.[6] The philosopher of science Ian Hacking points out that categories that originally represented a human state or a behavior are diverted into a category that represent a type of people. Hacking calls such categories "human kinds" (Hacking 1996). The title of this book shows that the term "hikikomori" refers to a type of people in such a condition.

Although Kudō did not directly define what hikikomori is, it is indicated as being those who are not "independent." Kudō defined independence as "having the power to lead one's life happily and in one's own way" (Kudō 1997, 140). Not having this power is the fundamental problem of hikikomori. According to Kudō, "a deep-rooted sense of 'shame' and culture also have a lot to do with the behavior of 'hikikomori'" (Kudō 1997, 42). In addition, "a sense of isolation and loneliness" (Kudō 1997, 42) and "devices to kill time," for example, NES, P.C., T.V., video, CD, and manga, make the hikikomori period prolonged (Kudō 1997, 43).

While Tomita defined hikikomori as a subjective experience, Kudō's perspective on hikikomori is based on his idea of "independence."[7] He believes that solution for the problem is to support hikikomori individuals to have a power to live their own lives, especially by earning their living. Since the 2000s, this context of "independence" in the sense of earning one's own living, becomes a keyword in social policy.

Japanese Journal of Clinical Psychiatry, Special Issue on the "Psychopathology of Hikikomori" (September 1997)

The September 1997 issue of the *Japanese Journal of Clinical Psychiatry* featured a special issue, "Psychopathology of Hikikomori." The term "hikikomori" here refers specifically to "non-psychotic hikikomori." In the opening article of the special issue, psychiatrists Sadanobu Ushijima and Jōji Satō wrote:

> Hikikomori has long been one of the most critical themes in psychiatry. . . . We have already intimately observed social isolation as a symptom of schizophrenic hikikomori, and hikikomori as the inhibition symptoms of depression. Therefore, some may question how much current significance there is in discussing hikikomori here and now, but on the other hand, it has become such an important theme that psychiatrists in general practice have never been more concerned with patients' "hikikomori" than they are today. There is no doubt that it has become an important theme. (Ushijima and Satō 1997, 1151)

According to Ushijima and Satō, contemporary hikikomori is a form of what Kasahara Yomishi calls *Taikyaku Shinkeishō* (withdrawal/retreat neurosis) a non-psychotic state of apathy, characterized by "total withdrawal from social life," a new and more severe form of *Taikyaku* (withdrawal/ retreat) (Ushijima and Satō 1997).[8] "Non-psychotic hikikomori" had become a problem for psychiatrists because those cases appeared in their practice. The later section will discuss this point.[9]

The opening article of the special issue of *Clinical Psychiatry* mentions two hikikomori cases. Both cases quit their jobs after graduating from university. The article interpreted these cases as instances of a "moratorium mentality" (i.e., attitudes that postpone the establishment of self-identity) that caused withdrawal from "external reality." This is an interpretation of hikikomori cases in a psychoanalytical context. It did not suggest any connection with school non-attendance, which some psychiatrists emphasized as being relevant to hikikomori.

Tamaki Saitō, Social Withdrawal: Adolescence without End (December 1998)

In December 1998, psychiatrist Tamaki Saitō published a book titled *Social Withdrawal: Adolescence without End [Shakaiteki Hikikomori: Owaranai*

Shishunki] (Saitō [1998] 2013).[10] This book is one of the most well-known
books on hikikomori in Japan. An English translation titled *HIKIKOMORI*
was published in 2013, and a new Japanese edition appeared in 2020. This
book as well as Saitō's exposure to the mass media as an expert on hikikomori
since the 2000s have contributed significantly to people's awareness of
hikikomori as a social problem (see chapter 2). Saitō himself states that he
wrote the book to raise awareness of the hikikomori problem and to generate
social interest (Saitō [1998] 2013, 12–13).

Saitō's framework for understanding the hikikomori problem is essential
in terms of its content and influence. He joined Hiroshi Inamura's laboratory
at the graduate school of Tsukuba University in 1986 and met *Shakaiteki
Hikikomori* adolescent cases. Saitō experienced more than 200 cases in the
10 years after that (Saitō [1998] 2013, 10–11).

Saitō defines hikikomori as a "state that has become a problem by the
late twenties, that involves cooping oneself up in one's own home and not
participating in society for six months or longer, but that does not seem to
have another psychological problem as its principal source" (Saitō [1998]
2013, 24). Although Saitō's definition is similar to other psychiatrists with
respect to mental disorder, what is unique about it is that he considers the
state of hikikomori itself as a problem and focused on this condition using the
term "social participation."[11] Saitō states, "the various symptoms associated
with social withdrawal are sometimes secondary," and he also insists that we
must think "the most continuous, stable, single symptom is the withdrawal
from society itself" (Saitō [1998] 2003, 26).[12]

The term "social participation" was familiar in the fields of education,
medical care, and social welfare in Japan. The field of education has used it
in phrases like "social participation of youth" since at least the late 1960s.
The fields of mental health and social welfare have also used this term in
phrases like "social participation of the disabled" since at least the 1980s.
Saitō's definition has positioned the hikikomori problem as a subject that
professionals from various fields can work on in concert. Since Saitō
proffered this definition, it has become common practice to approach the
hikikomori problem by way of "social participation."

As can be seen in the subtitle "Adolescence without End," Saitō considers
hikikomori to be a problem "deeply rooted in an adolescent mindset" which
arises "from the failure to mature as one travels along the path of character
development" (Saitō [1998] 2013, 28). Here, the hikikomori category is
associated with a failure to mature, and this point has a certain similarity
with Kudō's definition (1997), which regards independence as the referential
standard.

Saitō emphasized the necessity of medical treatment for hikikomori
cases and planned to establish the condition of hikikomori as a clinical unit

for intervention. He contended that people "who have been in a state of withdrawal for years and whose situations have grown chronic cannot recover without sufficient care from their family, as well as treatment by a specialist" (Saitō [1998] 2013, 94). Furthermore, he argued, "Should all people in social withdrawal be treated, regardless of whether they want to be or not? Let me jump right to my conclusion. I think that yes, people in withdrawal should be treated" (Saitō [1998] 2013, 99).[13]

Saitō actively promotes treatment because of the following circumstances surrounding hikikomori cases:

> There are a few unfortunate, overlapping factors that make the issue of social withdrawal so problematic. The first problem is that even though it is possible to prevent and treat it, there are hardly any facilities designed to do so. Families trying to deal with this problem typically have nowhere to turn to but a psychiatrist; however, psychiatrists tend to be halfhearted in dealing with the problem. (Saitō, [1998] 2013, 23)

Saitō also emphasized, "One cannot explain the problem of social withdrawal as merely the product of individual pathology" and "It is absolutely necessary to understand social withdrawal as a pathological system that involves both society and the family as well" (Saitō, [1998] 2013, 23). He describes this "pathological system" as a "hikikomori system," which refers to a communication deficiency among the individual, the family, and society. The smallest circle represents the individual in figure 4.1, the middle circle represents family, and the outermost circle represents society. This

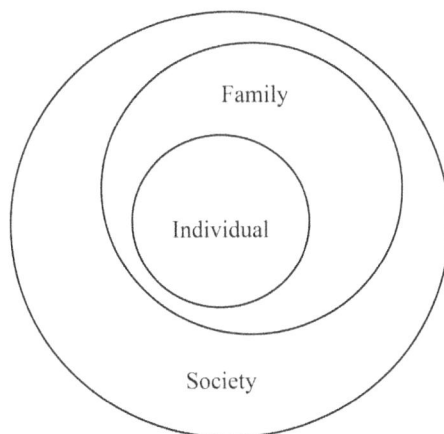

Figure 4.1   Model of Hikikomori System (Simplified Version of Saitō [1998] 2013, 84).
Source: Created by the author based on Saitō ([1998] 2013, 84).

figure explains that the hikikomori problem is a state in which "the points of contact have been cut off from one another" (Saitō [1998] 2013, 83).

Saitō noted that "the tendency to 'keep to oneself' on the part of the parents is characteristically Japanese" (Saitō [1998] 2013, 89). For Saitō, the essence of the hikikomori problem is the situation in which parents voluntarily keep to themselves and, at the same time, are forced to keep their hikikomori children to themselves because of lack of social support. His concept of the hikikomori system made it possible to view the various hikikomori cases "in an integrated manner" (Saitō 1998, 218).[14]

Although Saitō considered the hikikomori problem as "a failure to mature," he also insisted that this problem is not only individual pathology and that social intervention from psychiatry is required. His strategy to define this problem in terms of "social participation" was successful, and many subsequent definitions of hikikomori, including the governmental definition, followed it.

Summary of the Late 1990s

In the late 1990s, Sadatsugu Kudō and psychiatrist Tamaki Saitō each proposed a novel understanding of hikikomori cases. Although there is a difference between Kudō's emphasis on the "independence" as earning a living and Saitō's emphasis on spiritual "maturity," both understand hikikomori as a problem of human development. Saitō's approach to hikikomori, which identified the hikikomori problem as a lack of "social participation," guided following definitions and approaches to hikikomori problem. The withdrawal condition (lack of social participation) became the primary target of intervention. The concept of independence has also received wider attention since the 2000s.

NATIONWIDE ATTENTION: THE 2000S

The Early 2000s

There were three criminal incidents between the end of 1999 and the first half of 2000 in which Japanese mass media reported that young hikikomori people were suspects.[15] Hikikomori came to be widely regarded as a criminal risk as a result of media coverage of these three incidents. Tamaki Saitō frequently appeared in the mass media and conducted enlightenment activities to counteract the stereotype of hikikomori as a criminal risk.

This chapter examines (1) discussions by psychiatrists during this period; (2) the first guideline on hikikomori by the MHLW, published in 2003; and (3) the Youth Development Policy Outline by the government.

An Expanding Target of Psychiatry: Discussion by Psychiatrists

The concept of "non-schizophrenic hikikomori" caused some confusions and conflicts among psychiatrists. One psychiatrist, Ken Takaoka, even criticized it as "pseudo-psychiatry" (Takaoka 2001). On the other hand, Naoji Kondō called for a "practical stance" for dealing with hikikomori (Kondō 2001, 14). This emphasis on a "practical stance" suggests a great variety of hikikomori cases coming into the clinic, and psychiatrists having to deal with those cases using the existing diagnostic criteria.

It is also crucial to consider the expanding target area of mental health as a background of clinical confusions regarding hikikomori cases. Saitō's stance that psychiatrists should intervene in hikikomori cases was shared to some extent by psychiatrists in the early 2000s. The following statement by a psychiatrist suggests it:

> At present, there are no clinicians who regard hikikomori in general as a mental disorder. However, there is a growing recognition that with this problem psychiatry has a responsibility to intervene somehow, to some extent. As the fields of school mental health and occupational mental health expand, Japanese psychiatry breaks away from the rigid shackles of thought that only disease is subject to medical treatment and clinicians. (Shimizu 2003, 232)

Sociologist Tatsushi Ogino points out that, as with the citation above, psychiatry is extending its range to cases which are not diseases but subjects of therapeutic support (Ogino 2008b, 215). The trend of expanding the subjects of psychiatry beyond traditional psychiatric cases, both among psychiatrists and users, is one reason why various hikikomori cases began seeking help at clinics. Saitō's argument for psychiatric intervention into the hikikomori problem in the late 1990s contributed to this trend.

Thus, psychiatrists pursued two different directions: one direction was to treat hikikomori cases with the existing system of psychiatric diagnoses. The other direction is not to include hikikomori cases in the psychiatric diagnoses but to treat them as a mental health problem. These different directions develop further in psychiatric discourses in subsequent periods.

Ministry of Health, Labour and Welfare, the Guideline for Community Mental Health Activities Regarding Hikikomori, Focusing on People in their Teens and Twenties (July 2003)

In July 2003, the MHLW published the first official guideline on hikikomori, *the Guideline for Community Mental Health Activities Regarding Hikikomori, Focusing on People in their Teens and Twenties* [*Jūdai, Nijūdai wo chūshin to shita "Hikikomori" wo meguru Chiiki Hoken Katsudō no Gaidorain:*

Seishin Hoken Fukushi Sentā, Hokenjo, Shichōson de donoyōni Taiō suru ka] (MHLW 2003). This guideline is based on an MHLW study, "Research on the Nature of Intervention in Community Mental Health Activities" (principal investigator: psychiatrist Junichirō Itō), conducted from 2000 to 2002.

The guideline defines hikikomori as follows: "A state in which social participation has narrowed due to various factors, and a place for living outside the home, employment or schooling, has been lost over a long period" (Itō 2004, 3). This definition has many similarities with the definition by Tamaki Saitō (1998). For example, although the duration of "six months or more" is removed in favor of "over a long period," the core definition as a state of narrowed social participation and the reference to employment and schooling as specific examples of social participation are also similar to Saitō's definition (Saitō 2002).

In addition, this guideline emphasizes that hikikomori is neither a "diagnostic category" nor a "single disease unit" and that various factors—including biological, psychological, and social factors—are related to the hikikomori condition: "Hikikomori is not a diagnosis nor a single disorder unit. Furthermore, it does not occur with a single cause, e.g., bullying, family relationships, or disorder. Biological, psychological, and social factors are intertwined in various ways to create the phenomenon of hikikomori" (Itō 2004, 3). This guideline mainly calls for mental health services, such as public mental health welfare centers, although it mentions social factors (Itō 2004, 7).

As Ogino points out, the fact that the guideline "clearly positions 'hikikomori' as a subject of psychiatric treatment and mental health welfare has certainly increased the degree of 'medicalization'" (Ogino 2008b, 214). The guideline's request to enhance mental health services for hikikomori partly overlaps with the Council on Youth Affairs report in 1991, which mandated an integrated counseling place for hikikomori youth.

Government Discourse Regarding Youth Independence (in 2003)

In April 2003, the Cabinet Office, Ministry of Economy, Trade and Industry, MHLW, and Ministry of Education, Culture, Sports, Science and Technology launched the Council for Youth Independence and Challenge Strategy (*Wakamono Jiritu Chōsen Senryaku Kaigi*) with ministers from each ministry. In June, it announced the "Plan for Youth Independence and Challenge" (*Wakamono Jiritsu Chōsen Puran*), a proposal for "comprehensive human resource measures," which educational sociologist Michiko Miyamoto evaluated as the first comprehensive support plan for youth employment issues (Miyamoto 2015b, 23).

Although the term "hikikomori" does not appear in this plan, the plan mentions "the current situation of the number of *Freeters* increasing to about 200,000 and the number of unemployed and jobless youth increasing to about 100,000" (Council for Strategy for Independence and Challenge of Youth 2003, 4). These unemployed youth implicitly included hikikomori cases.

The government started to pay attention to youth employment in the first half of the 2000s in reaction to the expansion of employment problems since the late 1990s, which the previous chapter examined: an increase of youth who could not find a full-time job immediately after graduating from school, which the parental generation took for granted. The plan also points out that "the causes of youth problems should not be attributed only to youths themselves but should be addressed as problems of incompatibility of social systems such as education, human resource development, and employment" (Council for Youth Independence and Challenge Strategy 2003, 3).

Headquarters for the Promotion of Youth Development, The "National Youth Development Policy Outline" (December 2003)

In June 2003, the Cabinet Office established the Headquarters for the Promotion of Youth Development (*Seishōnen Ikusei Suishin Honbu*) and published the "National Youth Development Policy Outline" (*Seishōnen Ikusei Shisaku Taikō*) to promote "measures for the development of the next generation."[16] Most of the specific support measures for the social independence of youth presented by this policy outline are from the "Plan for Youth Independence and Challenge" mentioned earlier.

This policy outline mentions the hikikomori problem as one of the new problems youth face as a result of social changes, as follows:

Today, Japanese society is undergoing rapid changes in its demographic structure, with declining birthrates and an aging population. It is becoming increasingly information-oriented, internationalized, and consumer-centered, which has a significant impact on the environment of youth, including their families, schools, workplaces, communities, and places for information and consumption. Families are becoming smaller and more unstable as the number of siblings decreases, the number of divorced and remarried families increases, and the unmarried rate rises. The spread of the Internet has opened up new horizons of communication while diluting human relationships in the immediate group. While these changes in society have had a positive impact on the number of youth who are involved in volunteer work, international contributions, and entrepreneurship, they have also aggravated various problems such as juvenile delinquency, school non-attendance, hikikomori, and abuse, and have caused a delay in the social independence of youth as a significant new problem. (Headquarters for the Promotion of Youth Development 2003)

Although it seems that the hikikomori condition is an example of "a delay in the social independence," this is not the case. The hikikomori problem here is in youth mental health problems and not directly connected to a delay in social independence. This policy outline classes hikikomori with other problems as follows: "mental problems often seen in school-age and adolescent youth, such as school non-attendance, hikikomori, eating disorders, and sexually deviant behavior."

However, it is essential to examine the concept of social independence in this policy outline because the social independence of youth will become a critical context to discuss the hikikomori problem in the late 2000s. Independence, as understood in this policy outline, refers to the condition of youth who finish school and get jobs so as to no longer depend on their birth families. In a section titled "Support for Social Independence," this outline mandates that "support shall be provided so that youth can have employment, leave parental care, participate in public life, and lead independent lives as members of society." This policy outline proposed comprehensive measures to support youth's independence to address the delay in youth's social independence. Furthermore, "Basic Direction of Policies for Each Age Group," mentioned social measures to support youth independence. For example, "public rental housing systems and financing systems should be utilized so that young households can lead independent residential lives" (Youth Development Promotion Headquarters 2003). So, the independence of youth primarily means being independent of parental care by having employment, and it is easy to understand that the hikikomori problem became interpreted as a problem of independence in this context.

Summary of the Early 2000s

The first half of the 2000s saw the emergence of the context of social independence in addition to the context of mental health welfare carried over from the late 1990s. These two crucial contexts separately consider the hikikomori problem as a target of employment support and medical treatment. Although the youth independence matter was not clearly yet connected to the hikikomori problem at this point, it rapidly became connected to it from mid-2000s.

Yutaka Shiokura, a journalist for the nationwide newspaper *Asahi Shinbun*, who had been covering hikikomori since the 1990s, pointed out the following: Fujiya Tomita, a representative hikikomori proponent in the first half of the 1990s, "did not bring the issue of employment to the forefront."

In contrast, Tamaki Saitō and Sadatsugu Kudō, representatives in the second half of the 1990s and later, held "the attitude of emphasizing 'a sound argument' that adults should work." The latter argument shows "an increased compulsory character and emphasis on employment" (Shiokura 2002, 9–11). As will be confirmed below, this trend became even more apparent in the late 2000s with the government's policy of youth independence support, and employment support became the dominant context for hikikomori support in the late 2000s.

The Late 2000s

This section explores the process whereby the "NEET" policy expanded and incorporated the hikikomori problem into the context of the social independence of youth in the late 2000s. Specifically, this section will discuss (1) the debate and policy development surrounding NEET; (2) the Youth Development Headquarters' revised Youth Development Policy Outline (December 2008); and (3) the Child and Youth Development Support Promotion Act (July 2007).

Setting up Employment Support for Youth in the Late 2000s

Since the 2000s, youth employment has been attracting massive attention in Japan, and the initial problem was the increase in the number of youths who are aging as they continue to work as *Freeters* and other non-regular employees. Labor economist Yūji Genda, in a journal featuring the hikikomori issue in 2005, looks back on the period from the 1990s to the early 2000s as follows:

> Up until the 1990s, employment problems were always the problems of middle-aged and older people. In particular, a great deal of attention was paid to the issue of re-employment of middle-aged and older unemployed people who had lost their jobs due to so-called "restructuring," such as business reorganization, company bankruptcies, and mergers. However, in the 2000s, the trend changed, and attention began to focus on the youth employment issue, which had hardly even been considered until then. The unemployment rate for those in their teens and twenties rose sharply and remained at a high level, and the increase in the number of so-called *Freeters* or youth who continue to work as non-regular employees after graduating from school, which is estimated to be as high as two or four million, became a serious social problem. (Genda 2005, 44)

Genda recalls that, when he realized that there were hundreds of thousands of "youth who feel deeply hopeless about work" and about the fact that they were aging, he felt that "the hikikomori problem had become apparent in the labor market" (Genda 2005, 45).

Since the mid-2000s, Genda and Reiko Kosugi, a researcher at the Japan Institute for Labor Policy and Training (JILPT), have set NEETs rather than *Freeters* as the new employment policy target. The concept of NEET was imported from the United Kingdom. The Japanese NEET is a modified version of the original NEET ("Not in Education, Employment or Training") concept used in British youth policy since the 1990s.[17] NEET in the United Kingdom was a concept to illuminate youth's "social exclusion," which included unemployed youth. However, the Japanese NEET concept as introduced by Reiko Kosugi was to highlight not socially excluded youth but "those who are not participating in social activities and therefore may become a future cost to society and are not sufficiently activated by current employment support measures" (Kosugi 2004, 6). Kosugi's problem-setting was to position "NEETs" as "entities to be activated," which suppressed attention to the macro-social structure and the public services other than activation discussed in the previous chapter.

The government incorporated this concept of NEET into the national labor policy, and the MHLW launched the School for Youth Independence (*Wakamno Jiritu Juku*) project in 2005, which supplied a budget for employment support measures for NEETs. Although it was abolished in fiscal 2009 due to project sorting (*Jigyō Shiwake*) during short-term regime change between September 2009 and November 2012, a total budget of 42.3 billion yen (approximately 36.7 million US dollars) was allocated for the five years from fiscal 2005 to 2009. Furthermore, the Community Youth Support Station (*Chiiki Wakamono Sapōto Stēshon*) project, which began in fiscal 2006 and continues to be a central measure of the government's youth independence support program, had a total budget of over 260 billion yen (approximately 225.6 million US dollars) in 10 years. The total budget for these two projects, which aim for the social independence of youth, was already more than 300 billion yen (260.4 million US dollars) by fiscal 2015, and this policy trend has brought many organizations and support personnel for hikikomori cases to bear on NEETs.[18] This tendency has accelerated since the late 2000s.

Headquarters for the Promotion of Youth Development, the revised "National Youth Development Policy Outline" (December 2008)

In December 2008, the Headquarters for the Promotion of Youth Development revised the "National Youth Development Policy Outline" for the first time in five years. The revised policy outline expresses concerns about the increase in young workers with precarious employment, young unemployment, and the persistence of economic inequality, and it singles out these concerns as the motivating factors for the revision:

> The previous outline was formulated when Japan was suffering from a prolonged economic slump following the collapse of the bubble economy. The Japanese economy was forced to undergo severe structural reforms, and the effects of these reforms, especially on youth, were manifested in difficulty to find jobs for new graduates, rising unemployment rates, and unstable employment. In addition, the increase of income disparity and the decline in the family capacity to support their children have been pointed out. The economy has since turned to recovery, but the growth in income and consumption has been slower than the recovery in corporate performance, while the diversification of employment patterns has progressed further. In this context, the number of *Freeters* and NEETs remains high, and there are growing concerns about the risk that the various problems of children and youth interact with each other and become more complex, and that the economic gap widens and becomes fixed across generations. (Headquarters for the Promotion of Youth Development 2008, 1–2)

Based on these concerns, the revised policy outline emphasizes measures to support youth who face unemployment, unstable employment, and poverty.

The 2008 revised policy outline has clearly articulated the hikikomori problem in two ways: the mental health problem and the social independence problem regarding employment. On the one hand, the revised policy outline mentions "measures to deal with mental problems" in "measures to deal with school non-attendance and hikikomori," and also establishes a new section on "measures to deal with hikikomori," which clearly states that mental health welfare centers are responsible for dealing with this issue. These descriptions position the hikikomori problem as a mental health welfare issue, in line with the MHLW's 2003 guideline.[19] On the other hand, it also defines the hikikomori problem as one of independence and social participation. The section "Efforts to support youth with difficulties comprehensively" proposed measures for "youth with difficulties in independence and social participation, such as NEETs and hikikomori." Here, the revised policy outline treats NEETs and hikikomori in the same context.

Act on Promotion of Development and Support for Children and Youth (July 2009)

In July 2009, the Act on Promotion of Development and Support for Children and Youth (*Kodomo Wakamono Ikusei Shien Suishin Hō*) was enacted. As stated in Article 1 of Chapter 1, this Act aimed to "provide support for the healthy development of children and youth, to enable children and youth to have a smooth life in society, given the worsening environment surrounding children and youth and the serious problems of children and youth who experience difficulties in having a smooth life in society." Furthermore, the Act stipulates the responsibilities of the national government and local governments for the healthy development of children and youth. This was the first Act that clarified the national and local governments' responsibility to support children and youth who "experience difficulties in having a smooth life in society."

Although the term "hikikomori" does not appear in this Act, Article 2 of Chapter 1 states that "the government shall provide the necessary support to children and youth who are neither studying nor working and who experience difficulties in having a smooth life in society." It is obvious that those children and youth include hikikomori cases.[20] This Act seeks to address the comprehensive difficulties faced by children and youth, and it calls for a social support system that includes various fields of education, medical care, and employment support.[21] It prepared the broader context—including mental health, employment support and social welfare—to treat the hikikomori problem.

Summary of the Late 2000s

It was only during the latter half of the 2000s when the social independence of youth and corresponding measures to support youth employment expanded rapidly implemented by the government. The Act for the Promotion of Support for Children and Youth Development also made it a public responsibility to support "children and youth who experience difficulties in having a smooth life in society," which would include the hikikomori problem.

The program to support youth employment was a breakthrough, because it was the first public support measures targeting young people who up until then had been ignored by social policy. However, the expenditure was limited to subsidizing employment support programs and there was still no menu of social benefits for youth.

THE CHANGING FRAMEWORK: IN THE 2010S

The Early 2010s

The Cabinet Office and the MHLW respectively published guidebooks on support for hikikomori cases in the 2010s, as did many local governments. This section will focus on (1) the MHLW's new guideline titled "Guidelines for the Evaluation and Support of Hikikomori," (2) the Cabinet Office's nationwide survey on hikikomori cases, (3) "Vision for Children and

Youth," (4) the Cabinet Office's *Handbook for Hikikomori Support People*, (5) the report on those in need by the Special Committee of the Social Security Council, and (6) the Act for Supporting the Independence of Those in Need.

Ministry of Health, Labor and Welfare, the Guideline for the Evaluation and Support of Hikikomori (May 2010)

The MHLW published a new guideline for hikikomori support, the *Guideline for the Evaluation and Support of Hikikomori* (*Hikikomori no Hyōka to Shien ni kansuru Guidorain*) based on its science research, "Actual Condition of Psychiatric Disorders Causing Adolescent Hikikomori and the Construction of a Psychiatric Treatment and Assistance System," conducted from 2007 to 2009, and it replaced the previous guideline published in 2003. The principal investigator of this research was child psychiatrist Kazuhiko Saitō, and the research team consisted mainly of psychiatrists, including Naoji Kondō and Tamaki Saitō.

This new guideline defines the hikikomori phenomenon as a non-psychotic phenomenon but emphasizes that schizophrenic cases are potentially included:

> A phenomenal concept that refers to a state in which a person avoids social participation (e.g., schooling including compulsory education, employment including part-time jobs, socializing outside the home) as a result of a variety of factors and, in principle, remains mainly at home for six months or more (even when going out in a way that does not involve interaction with others). In principle, hikikomori is a non-psychotic phenomenon distinct from hikikomori based on positive or negative symptoms of schizophrenia, but it should be noted that it is not unlikely to include schizophrenia before a definitive diagnosis is made. (MHLW 2010)

Compared to the previous guideline, this new guideline emphasizes the connection of the hikikomori with school non-attendance and NEET problems, and it further attempts to incorporate hikikomori into the existing mental disorder categories.[22] This new guideline refers to a study by Kondō and his colleagues (Kondō et al. 2010), which found that almost all cases of hikikomori consultations at mental health welfare centers received diagnoses of mental disorders.[23] This new guideline states that mental health, welfare, and medical treatment are essential to treat hikikomori cases. However, it proposes psychiatric diagnoses of hikikomori cases in detail and aims to develop a comprehensive psychiatric treatment for the hikikomori problem.

The Cabinet Office, Survey Report on Youth Consciousness
(Fact-Finding Survey on Hikikomori) (July 2010)

In July 2010, the Cabinet Office released the report of its nationwide survey on hikikomori, *Survey Report on Youth Consciousness.* The report put the incidence of hikikomori cases at 1.79% among the population aged 15 to 39 years old, and it estimated nearly 696,000 hikikomori cases among the same age group in Japan (Cabinet Office 2010). The national newspapers reported this estimated number widely (e.g., Yomiuri Shinbun, July 24, 2010, morning edition). This survey excludes mental disorder cases from the hikikomori group, defining the hikikomori condition as applying only to those who have been living mainly at home for six months or more, and whose reasons for doing so are not "schizophrenia, physical illness, pregnancy, working at home, childbirth, childcare, or housework."[24]

There is a clear difference in views on hikikomori between the MHLW guideline and the Cabinet Office survey report. While the new MHLW guideline considered that diagnoses of mental disorders could include most of the hikikomori cases, in contrast the Cabinet Office survey report excluded schizophrenia cases from the hikikomori group. Psychiatrist Takehiko Yoshikawa, who was involved in the design and analysis of this hikikomori survey, criticized the MHLW's new guidelines as follows:

> Japanese society has regarded hikikomori as if it were a specific condition caused by psychopathological factors and has conducted surveys to get the answer that "psychiatric or mental health methods should treat this hikikomori." Moreover, we should consider the bias in survey objects because they had to resort to obtaining survey targets through "mental health-related facilities" such as public health centers and mental health welfare centers because of the difficulty in obtaining survey samples. (Yoshikawa 2010, 32)

This criticism highlights a significant difference of opinion among psychiatrists, and also between the MHLW and the Cabinet Office, regarding the medicalization of hikikomori cases. The MHLW guideline aims to advance the medicalization of hikikomori cases by including them in the current diagnoses. In contrast, Yoshikawa does not try to include hikikomori as a psychiatric diagnosis but treats it as a mental health issue. These different stances are probably related to members of the planning and analysis council of this survey. Four of them (including the chairman) were psychologists, and one (Yoshikawa) was a psychiatrist. In contrast, 11 of the 13 research fellows of the MHLW guideline (including the principal investigator) were psychiatrists, while the other two were a clinical psychologist and a dentist (specializing in public health).

Another feature of this survey is that it included cases who can leave their homes in the hikikomori group, and the ratio of the cases that cannot leave home is 11.9% among the hikikomori group. As for the frequency of leaving home among the 59 hikikomori cases, the distribution is the following: 66.1% "only go out when they have something related to their hobbies"; 22.0% "usually stay at home but go out to, e.g., the local convenience store"; 5.1% "go out from their own room but not from home"; 6.8% "rarely go out from their own room." If the survey had defined hikikomori as only those who never actually left home, the number of cases would have been much smaller.

The Cabinet Office states that the reason for this approach was to "focus on whether or not the person has reached social independence." This statement suggests that the Cabinet Office understands the hikikomori problem as being related to employment and independence from parents. Thus, this report assumes an employment context of the hikikomori problem and it estimates a fairly wide range of hikikomori cases, including those who are able to leave home. Although defining hikikomori in this way remained controversial, the inclusion of those who can leave home in this report succeeded in impressing people with the considerable number of hikikomori cases.

Headquarters for the Promotion of Support for the Development of Children and Youth, "Vision for Children and Youth" (July 2010)

In July 2010, the Headquarters for the Promotion of Support for the Development of Children and Youth published a policy outline titled "Vision for Children and Youth" (*Kodomo Wakamono Bijon*).[25] This policy outline came under the "Act for the Promotion of Support for the Development of Children and Youth" enacted in 2009, and it replaced the "Policy Outline for Youth Development" enacted in 2008. The Democratic Party of Japan (DPJ) established this policy outline during its short time in power, from September 2009 until November 2012.

The beginning of this policy outline declared that the national government, local governments, and private organizations would work together on measures for the development of children and youth, based on the principles of the Act:

> The measures for supporting the development of children and youth cover almost every field of society, including education, welfare, health, medical care, correction, rehabilitation, and employment. We will do our utmost to address this issue with close cooperation among the relevant national and local government agencies, private organizations, and others. (Headquarters for the Promotion of Support for the Development of Children and Youth 2010)[26]

This policy outline mentions hikikomori in a passage titled "Efforts to support children and youth with difficulties and their families":

> There are children and youth who have special needs due to various difficulties. The problems widely range from difficulties in having a smooth life in society, such as NEET, hikikomori and school non-attendance, to disabilities, suffering from crime, including abuse, and being a long-term foreign resident in Japan. We will provide the support each difficulty requires. For children and youth who have fallen into delinquency or crime, we consider their difficulties and support them to recover as members of society. We provide support not only to the children and youth themselves but also to their families. We will also proactively address the issue of child poverty. (Headquarters for the Promotion of Support for the Development of Children and Youth 2010)

This perspective achieves a broader concept of children and youth who experience "difficulties in having a smooth life in society," and it includes hikikomori explicitly here.

This policy outline also mentions the Hikikomori Community Support Center (*Hikikomori Chiiki Sapōto Sentā*) as a primary consultation center for the hikikomori problem. This is an achievement by the KHJ, which lobbied to establish a special institute to support hikikomori cases.[27] This policy outline also states that vocational independence will be promoted through a Community Youth Support Station (*Chiiki Wakamono Sapōto Sutēshon*) project for NEETs and other youth.[28]

This policy outline relates the hikikomori problem with social independence indirectly by mentioning a community youth support station for employment support, but it does not use the term "independence." Rather, this policy outline promotes a stance not exclusively focusing on employment support, but emphasizing broader or multifaceted support for a "smooth social life."

The Cabinet Office Handbook for Hikikomori Support People (July 2011)

In July 2011, the Cabinet Office published the *Handbook for Hikikomori Support People* (Cabinet Office 2011) and distributed it to relevant organizations nationwide. The handbook contains contributions from a variety of specialists, psychiatrists, a psychosomatic physician, a career counselor, a mental health worker, and a financial planner.

However, the Cabinet Office did not make any comment on how to define the hikikomori problem and how to treat the problem in the handbook. The Cabinet Office's original statement is only one page, "On Publication." It points out that hikikomori cases have become protracted, and it concludes,

"We hope that the circle of social support will expand even further." It is in contrast to the MHLW, which was actively pursuing a policy of medicalizing hikikomori.

Without the explicit standpoint of the Cabinet Office, some contributors stress the importance of self-help for family members. For example, a financial planner insists on the necessity for parents to have a financial "survival plan." This handbook gave families with hikikomori children an impression of the significance of the "self-responsibility" of parents or the "family responsibility" for the hikikomori problem. A woman with a hikikomori son in his mid-twenties wrote her impressions of this handbook as follows:

> Recently, I had a chance to read the *Handbook for Hikikomori Support People* published by the Cabinet Office. The book seemed to focus on "developmental disability" as the cause [of hikikomori cases]. On the other hand, it explains in a "careful and detailed" manner, even bringing in a financial planner, that it will be manageable if the parents are responsible for spending all their assets without relying on the social security system when the condition of hikikomori or inability to fend for oneself becomes prolonged. I could not help but feel that both of these were trying to sweep away the hikikomori problem with the "self-responsibility" of the parents and the hikikomori subjects. As a parent of one, I cannot help but feel doubtful and angry. (Aoki et al. 2015, 31)

This handbook did not show any unified understanding of the hikikomori problem. However, as this woman suggested, it had a hidden assumption of family self-help and implies that families with hikikomori children must treat the problem by themselves.

The Social Security Council, Report of Special Subcommittee on Livelihood Support for Those in Need (January 2013)

The special subcommittee of the Social Security Council on Livelihood Support for Those in Need (*Shakai Hoshō Shingikai, Seikatsu Konkyūsha no Seikatsu Shien no Arikata ni kansuru Tokubetsu Bukai*) was established in April 2012 under the DPJ administration to "consider measures for those in need and review the public assistance system in an integrated manner" in response to the "increase in the number of those in need and public assistance recipients."

Under "Prevention of Poverty among Children and Youth" in the section "Construction of a New Support System for Those in Need," this report refers to hikikomori in the following way:

> The problems faced by children and youth have become increasingly severe and complex in recent years. Due to family poverty, parental divorce, or family

disintegration, there are children and youth who cannot get the support which they need to become independent from their parents, have significant problems with low academic achievement and communication skills, and cannot obtain opportunities for education and training; they fail at everything and accumulate experience of failures after they go out into society and become NEET and hikikomori. (Social Security Council 2013, 32)

The purpose of this report is to address how to prevent poverty in order to reduce the number of public-assistance recipients, and it is the first time that the hikikomori problem appeared in an administrative document in the context of social welfare for poverty-prevention explicitly. This report places hikikomori cases in the context of those in need and, more specifically, in the context of future public-assistance recipients. The report suggests that NEET and hikikomori are part of the vicious cycle of poverty and stresses the need for social support to prevent poverty.[29] This report emphasizes the hikikomori problem in terms of social welfare policy, and its framework is different from previous ones, which placed the problem in the contexts of mental health welfare (medical treatment) and social independence (employment support).

Act for Supporting the Independence of Those in Need (December 2013)

Based on the 2013 report by the special subcommittee of the Social Security Council, the Act for Supporting the Independence of Those in Need (*Seikatsu Konkyūsha Jiritsu Shien Hō*) was enacted in December 2013. Following that, the System for Supporting the Independence of Those in Need (*Seikatsu Konkyūsha Jiritsu Shien Seido*) started in April 2015. The Act defines the concept of "those in need" (*Seikatsu Konkyūsha*) as "persons who are actually in financial need and are likely to become unable to maintain a minimum standard of living."

The MHLW website, which explains this system, includes the following sentence for background: "In recent years, as the socioeconomic environment has changed, the number of welfare recipients, including those at high risk of becoming impoverished and those of working age, has increased. In order to respond to this situation, comprehensive efforts are currently being made to establish a new support system for those in need and to review the public assistance system" (MHLW 2022a).

The new support system provides a support person who prepares an individual support plan according to the client's needs. It also provides such services as housing security assistance, employment preparation support, household budget consultation, training for employment, study support for children from households in need, and temporary living support (MHLW 2022b).

The primary purpose of the new support system is to prevent poverty before an individual receives public assistance, and the "independence" in the Act has an additional meaning to the term previously mentioned. In the context of employment support, it means independence from family. However, here this term also signifies independence from public assistance. As a measure for that, this new system provides "comprehensive support," including a personal support plan and housing support.

The MHLW published a leaflet that introduced the new system and describes "Mr. A (38 years old, male), a case of long-term hikikomori" (MHLW 2015). After dropping out of high school, Mr. A lived by taking care of his mother while relying on his father's (age 80) welfare pension. With the support of a social worker from the support system, he became employed, and his mother could use the nursing care insurance system instead.

The hikikomori problem discussed here is not only in the context of social independence (i.e., employment support), a context that had persisted since the 1990s and which assumed inclusion in a stable male-breadwinner system, but also poverty-prevention, which newly emerged as a context to discuss families with hikikomori cases (See also MHLW 2018). However, this system offers very little in the way of benefits for users; the main purpose of this system is to provide services to prevent people from being dependent on the public assistance.

Summary of the Early 2010s

Since the latter half of the 2000s, the hikikomori category has been combined with the NEET category as a target of employment support. At the same time, the hikikomori category was a target of mental health welfare—although there are differences of opinion among psychiatrists focused on the hikikomori problem. Thus, two main streams of support for hikikomori cases were established: employment support and mental health welfare.

However, the hikikomori problem was discussed in the context of poverty prevention from the mid-2010s, which did not exclude the contexts of employment support and mental health welfare, but rather positioned the problem in the context of social welfare policy and maintenance of the public-assistance system. Considering that the hikikomori problem appeared at the end of the 1980s as a "psychological problem created by material affluence," the transformation of the framework for understanding the hikikomori problem over the past 20 years is astounding.

The Late 2010s

In the late 2010s, the hikikomori issue was increasingly discussed in the context of social welfare policy. This section treats (1) the national survey of hikikomori in 2015, (2) the revised "Policy Outline for Children and Youth Development" in 2016, (3) the national survey of middle-aged hikikomori cases in 2017, (4) the revision of the Social Welfare Act, and (5) criminal cases related to hikikomori and the subsequent announcement by the MHLW.

The Cabinet Office, Survey Report on Youth Living (September 2016)

The Cabinet Office surveyed the hikikomori in December 2015 and published a report in September 2016. The research design was almost the same as the 2010 survey. The report put incidents of hikikomori cases among 15–39-year-olds at 1.57%, and it estimated the number of hikikomori cases as 541,000 (Cabinet Office 2016). One of the nationwide newspapers, *Asahi Shinbun*, reported the survey results under the heading "Hikikomori 540,000 in ages 15 to 39, a prolonged trend, the Cabinet Office estimates" on September 9, 2016. According to that article, "In terms of the period of hikikomori, the largest percentage, 34.7%, gave the response of more than seven years. This number has doubled from 16.9% in the previous survey. Regarding the age at which they became hikikomori, more than 60% of the respondents chose the age range 15–24, and they gave reasons such as 'not attending school' or 'not fitting in at work.' 10.2% of the respondents chose the age range 35–39, and this percentage is up from 5.1% in the previous survey" (*Asahi Shinbun*, September 9, 2016, morning edition). A different version of this article on the *Asahi Shinbun* website cites the following comment from a Cabinet Office official: "We would like to provide support through consultation services and other institutions so that the situation can be improved in a short period and, for example, lead to employment."

Among the 49 hikikomori cases, the percentage of those who never left the house was only 10.2%. The response regarding the behavior of going out was the following: 67.3% "only go out when they have to do something related to their hobbies"; 22.4% "usually stay at home but go out to the local convenience store"; 10.2% "go out from their own room but not from home"; 0.0% "rarely go out from their own room." As in the 2010 Cabinet Office survey report, the majority of hikikomori cases in this study are able to leave home.

The Cabinet Office did not change the hikikomori definition, which "focuses on whether or not the person has reached social independence." As with the 2010 survey, it kept defining hikikomori cases from the perspective of social independence, which includes many hikikomori cases that leave home. The report also showed the prolonged tendency and aging of subjects, as the comment of the Cabinet Office official suggests.

Headquarters for the Promotion of Support for the Development of Children and Youth, the "Policy Outline for the Promotion of Support for Children and Youth Development" (February 2016)

In February 2016, the "Vision for Children and Youth" was revised as the "Policy Outline for the Promotion of Support for Children and Youth Development" (*Kodomo Wakamono Ikusei Shien Suishin Taikō*) by the Liberal Democratic Party, which returned to power from December 2012. While the previous Policy Outline focused on an inclusive society, the new Policy Outline focused on "the independence and activities of children and youth" (Headquarters for Promoting Support for Children and Youth Development 2016).[30]

However, the treatment for hikikomori in the new Policy Outline did not change that much from the previous Policy Outline of 2010. The new Policy Outline states that "primary consultation centers for hikikomori, community support centers for hikikomori, mental health welfare centers, public health centers, municipal health centers, and child guidance centers provide consultation and support" (Headquarters for the Promotion of Support for the Development of Children and Youth 2016).

The Cabinet Office, Survey Report on Living Conditions (March 2019)

In December 2018, the Cabinet Office conducted a new hikikomori survey which targeted the older age group from 40 to 64 years old (Cabinet Office 2019). The following year's *White Paper on Children and Youth* featured the survey results as a special issue under the title, "The reality of prolonged hikikomori." This special issue focuses on the following points of the survey results: (1) the incidence of hikikomori in the age group of 40–64-year-olds is 1.45%, and the estimated number is 613,000. (2) About 50% of the respondents have been hikikomori for more than seven years, indicating a tendency to stay hikikomori for an extended period. (3) There are also hikikomori cases of housewives and homeworkers. (4) The prevalence of hikikomori is distributed evenly across all age groups (Cabinet Office 2019b).

The percentage of those who did not leave home was 14.9% among the 47 hikikomori cases because the definition of hikikomori in this survey continued to construct the hikikomori problem focusing on "social independence" (Cabinet Office 2019a, 9). This definition has a gap from the stereotypical image of hikikomori, which means the condition of not going out from their rooms or houses. Nevertheless, mass media rarely focused on the fact that the majority of hikikomori cases can and do go out, but they reported an estimate that there are more than 1 million hikikomori cases when added to the result of the 2016 survey.

In addition, a few years before this survey result, the term "80 50 problem [*Hachimaru Gōmaru Mondai*]" had become known; it means parents in their 80s taking care of their hikikomori children in their 50s.[31] This term spread widely with the Cabinet Office survey result by mass media reports (*Asahi Shinbun*, March 29, 2019, evening edition; May 13, 2020, morning edition).

Revision of the Social Welfare Act (May 2017)

Parliament amended the Social Welfare Act (*Shakai Fukushi Hō*) in May 2017 in order to codify the concept of the *community-inclusive society* (*Chiiki Kyōsei Shakai*), which means a society in which local government and residents together proactively produce the community welfare, indicated in the Japan All Active Plan (*Nippon Ichioku Sō Katsuyaku Puran*) approved by the Cabinet in 2016.

The amended Act states that municipalities are responsible for promoting community welfare in cooperation with community residents. In particular, it stipulates: (1) the aim to achieve solutions to community problems through comprehension and cooperation by residents, those involved in welfare, and institutions; (2) that the municipality shall make efforts to establish a comprehensive support system to achieve that aim; and (3) a focus on the enhancement of community welfare planning (Hashikawa 2021).

Further amendments to the Social Welfare Act were made in 2020. In this context, the concept of a community-inclusive society positioned the hikikomori problem as an issue relegated to the margins of the existing social welfare system, and the MHLW emphasized that community welfare must support the social participation of hikikomori cases through comprehensive consultation (MHLW 2019b).

Kawasaki City Child Murder Case, Nerima Ward Son Murder Case, and the MHLW Announcement (May–June 2019)

On May 28, 2019, in Kawasaki City, Kanagawa Prefecture, a 51-year-old man with a kitchen knife attacked a line of children waiting for a school bus for a private elementary school. He killed a father, who had come to see his child off, and another child, and injured 18 others. The attacker committed suicide by stabbing himself in the neck on the spot. News articles reported that the man had been living with his aunt and her husband after his parents divorced and that he had been hikikomori for more than ten years before the crime (*Asahi Shinbun*, June 4, 2019 morning edition; June 28, 2019 morning edition).

Four days after this incident, in Nerima Ward, Tokyo, a 77-year-old man, a former vice-minister of the Ministry of Agriculture, Forestry and Fisheries, stabbed his 44-year-old son to death. A news article reported that the son had been hikikomori for many years and had a history of domestic violence. Just before the crime, the son started saying "I will kill them" in response to a Sports Day at an elementary school next to his house, which reminded the father of the incident in Kawasaki City, so he decided to kill his son (*Asahi Shinbun*, June 4, 2019, morning edition).

In response to these incidents, the minister of MHLW, Takumi Nemoto, issued the following message on June 26, 2019: "All those in a state of hikikomori and their families have different backgrounds and circumstances. We need to take the time to support them as they struggle daily with the difficulties of life and isolation. . . . I would like to ask for the understanding and cooperation of all citizens in realizing a mighty community-inclusive society in which all people can live together, without isolation, and with roles to play" (MHLW 2019a).[32] The minister of MHLW also mentioned the 80 50 problem after mentioning these criminal cases (*Asahi Shinbun*, June 4, 2019, evening edition). The MHLW emphasized that the community-inclusive society must play an essential role in solving the hikikomori problem, as with the 80 50 problem (*Asahi Shinbun*, May 13, 2020, morning edition). Through the minister's announcements and these news reports, the hikikomori problem became more deeply incorporated into the context of the 80 50 problem and the community-inclusive society.

Summary of the Late 2010s

The late 2010s was a period in which the hikikomori problem attracted enormous attention in Japanese society. Middle-aged or elderly hikikomori cases received attention through the survey report by the cabinet office, and the 80 50 problem became crucial in the discourses which discussed the hikikomori problem in this period. The context of social welfare developed from reducing public-assistance recipients in the early 2010s toward a community-inclusive society policy, which reinforces family and community responsibility under the vector of the Finance Ministry's constraint on social security expenditure.

CONSIDERATIONS: THE FUTURE OF
THE HIKIKOMORI PROBLEM

Three Contexts of Hikikomori Discourse

This chapter has confirmed three significant contexts since the late 2000s in discussing hikikomori. First, the context of social independence, which assumes employment (integration into labor market) as a solution. The main measures in this context are employment support and career consultation. Second, the context of social welfare, which focuses on poverty prevention and social isolation. Third, the context of mental health, which assumes mental health maintenance by psychiatry as a solution to the problem. This third context includes two different stances; one aims to include hikikomori cases in the psychiatric system of diagnoses, and the other aims to treat hikikomori cases as a mental health issue without psychiatric diagnoses.

While the third context of mental health focuses mainly on the behavior and psychology of the individual, the first and second contexts are both related to the issue of life security discussed in chapter 3. The first context of social independence basically refers to independence from the family through the achievement of employment (inclusion in corporate welfare), which is also the basis for the definition of "hikikomori" in the Cabinet Office surveys. Since the 2010s, a new meaning has been added to the concept of independence related to hikikomori in the context of social welfare. This is indicated by the title of the "Act for Supporting the Independence of Those in Need" (*Seikatsu Konkyūsha Jiritsu Shien Hō*) established in December 2013. The concept of independence in this context of poverty prevention has the implication of not being dependent on the welfare state, especially public assistance, because the context of poverty prevention connotes preventing the family unit's dependence on public assistance in order to protect the public-assistance system from an increasing number of recipients (Katada 2017). In other words, "independence" in the context of social welfare has a dual meaning: social independence as independence from the family through employment, and independence from the welfare state.

These three contexts need to be distinguished from each other; however, they are also complementary in the discourses of the hikikomori problem. For example, the MHLW guideline in 2010 considered employment supports as the next step in mental health treatment. The "System for Supporting the Independence of Those in Need" (*Seikatsu Konkyūsha Jiritsu Shien Seido*) provides employment support in order to achieve both independence from family and the public assistance.[33]

The first and second contexts, which share the issue of life security, will be discussed together in the next section. Then the third context, that of mental health, will be examined.

Hikikomori in the Employment and Social Welfare Contexts

The government has considered employment support an essential measure to treat the social-independence-from-family problem since the 2000s, given the increase in non-regular employment and unemployment, especially among youth. However, the direction of solving the hikikomori problem through support for full-time employment, which assumes the male-breadwinner model, has come to an impasse (Miyamoto 2015a, 20–24).[34]

Since the 2010s, the context of social welfare has moved into the foreground in discourses on hikikomori. One of the reasons for this change is that it has become challenging to assume the model of life security by inclusion in corporate welfare. In addition, the increased attention paid to aged hikikomori cases and the 80 50 problem has also accelerated this change of problem recognition.

The poverty-prevention context emerged in response to the shrinking inclusivity of corporate welfare and the 80 50 problem. The "System for Supporting the Independence of Those in Need" since 2015 has provided social services to prevent poverty. However, though this support system for those in need provides financial support for housing, that is not fully effective because of a limited benefit period of three months and a severe restriction based on annual household income. In order to prevent public-assistance dependency, the poverty-prevention seeks to leverage family resources to take care of jobless family members, as well as to support employment.

This social welfare context has merged with the wider context of a community-inclusive society in the late 2010s, which focuses on community inclusion to treat the problems of isolation and poverty. However, this focus on a community-inclusive society has been criticized by many scholars. Hashikawa (2021) singled out as representative the criticisms of Yamazaki (2019) and Miyamoto (2017). According to Mitsuhiro Yamazaki of the Japan Center for the Disabled (*Nihon Shōgaisha Sentā*), this policy concept aims to regress public responsibility for social security and social welfare, because it goes back to the Japanese-style welfare society policy that aimed to enhance welfare based on families and communities (Yamazaki 2019, 9–10). According to Tarō Miyamoto, two vectors are at work in the vision of a community-inclusive society: one vector is to realize better and more comprehensive services that meet people's needs and to create employment opportunities and places people can belong to in community, and the other vector is to cut social security expenditure from fiscal authorities by emphasizing the community responsibility (Miyamoto 2017, 10–11). As these scholars appear to point out correctly that the social welfare policy of a community-inclusive society can diminish public welfare by emphasizing community mutual aid.[35]

It seems impossible that the community welfare could cover all the people in need, at least without financial backing, in place of diminishing corporate welfare and unstable family welfare. These two contexts together raise a question: how hikikomori adult children can become independent from their families and at the same time not dependent on the welfare state.

Such a question is unlikely to be solved by simply advocating the idea of the community-inclusive society.

Hikikomori as a Mental Health Problem

According to Peter Conrad and Joseph W. Schneider (Conrad and Schneider 1992), to define a problem in medical terms (usually as a disease or disorder) is to assert that the medical professional is a legitimate expert in dealing with that problem. Thus, what is at stake in the debate over whether or not hikikomori is subject to psychiatric treatment is a debate about the legitimate authority to define and hold social control over the hikikomori problem.[36]

Even though the MHLW released a guideline in 2010, which claimed that the current diagnoses of mental disorders could include most of the hikikomori cases, the hikikomori problem remains within a broader context of mental health, employment support, and social welfare.

There are several reasons for this situation where there is still no one authority to treat the hikikomori problem. One of the reasons, as this chapter has examined, is that the contexts of hikikomori discourse is plural, and the mental health context cannot cover the social independence and social welfare contexts. Another reason, as the previous chapter discussed, is that the maximum responsibility of family for taking care of hikikomori cases. Other systems (like the mental health care system, community youth support center, and hikikomori community support center) have just been supplementary and have never taken the place of family responsibility. Disability pensions also do not cover hikikomori cases well enough. Thus, psychiatric professionals cannot offer adequate life security for hikikomori cases in place of their families. This situation does not allow psychiatry to be exclusive authority to deal with the hikikomori problem.

Psychiatry has no exclusive authority—but this, as a result, avoids the individualization of the hikikomori problem. As Conrad and Schneider point out, medicalization can have a consequence for society by reducing deviance to individual pathology (Conrad and Schneider 1992, 250), so that medicalization of the hikikomori problem diminishes social aspects of that problem. The lack of exclusive psychiatric authority of this problem also means that there is multifaceted support for hikikomori cases. Psychiatrist Tamaki Saitō welcomes this situation:

> In my opinion, non-medical support has achieved a lot in the field of supporting hikikomori until now. Promoting medicalization unnecessarily, without a certain amount of respect for their "expertise" and collaboration with them [non-medical support professionals], may reduce the potential of already scarce social resources. At this point, psychiatrists require a humble acceptance that

therapeutic support is only one effective means of support and is complementary to traditional [non-psychiatric] support. (Saitō 2015, 1567)

While there are desirable aspects when no single authority has control to treat the hikikomori problem, it would not necessarily be desirable, however, to have a diverse set of contexts mixed in an unorganized manner. This chapter showed that there are at least three major contexts since the late 2000s: social independence from family, social welfare (especially poverty prevention), and mental health. It is necessary to understand the discourse on the hikikomori problem by grasping the framework used to understand the problem: who sees what as the hikikomori problem, and which solutions are proposed for it.

CONCLUSION

This chapter clarified the significant transformation of contexts in discourses concerning the hikikomori problem. In the late 1980s, a few discourses started to explore the hikikomori problem. In the 1990s, governmental discourses considered the hikikomori problem as one of "asocial" behavior. In the 2000s, government discourse identified hikikomori within two contexts: (1) social independence, which assumed integration into corporate welfare; and (2) a mental health issue, which psychiatry could treat. Until the 2010s, those discourses assumed that family welfare was fully responsible for supporting hikikomori cases.

However, since the 2010s, governmental discourses could not keep assuming family welfare as an inclusive resource for children excluded from corporate welfare. Consequently, the concept of the community-inclusive society emerged, designating the community as a new actor to support those in need. This new expectation of community support for hikikomori cases is a development in the Japanese style of welfare society policy, which has left life-security functions to the private sector.

The changing contexts of hikikomori discourses suggest a transformation of Japanese society since the end of the 1980s. Thus, those discourses can be a touchstone to explore how the future Japanese society could construct or fail to construct a genuinely inclusive system for isolated individuals.

NOTES

1. Kitao's definition of "emotional disorders" is low self-esteem and feelings of inferiority (Kitao 1986: 38).
2. The editor of this book, behavior therapist Shigeo Kobayashi, considers hikikomori to be an individual behavioral problem of each child. The "social

withdrawal" (*shakaiteki hikikomori*) behavior prevents the child from having opportunities to master social skills, which in turn hampers nursing, childcare, and educational achievements, and also induces in the child personality and behavioral conditions that can lead to their being bullied, school refusal, and selective silence. Thus, "in some cases, this state [of hikikomori] persists into late adolescence. If these symptoms of hikikomori are not resolved as soon as possible, they may lead to various accompanying problems" (Kobayashi 1989).

3. Psychiatrist Saitō Tamaki mentions in his 1998 book that this project excludes over 90% of hikikomori cases who are over 18 years old (Saitō [1998] 2003, 177).

4. This project has three main programs: (1) the Spiritual Friend (*Mentaru Furendo*) dispatching program, which deploys university students who have passion for child welfare to homes with a hikikomori child; (2) the lodging with guidance and support program, which accommodates children in child facilities and includes them in group activities; and (3) the liaison conference on welfare and education for children, which coordinates institutions involved in child welfare and education (e.g., child guidance centers, schools, public health centers) (Uchida 2005).

5. The report identified six factors contributing to the increase in asocial problem behaviors: (1) socioeconomic changes (e.g., loss of living attitudes amid convenience, a decline in the educational function of local communities), (2) changes in social consciousness (e.g., materialistic values, the prevalence of middle-class consciousness, sense of being able to see what is to come), (3) the current state of the family (e.g., changes in the educational function of the family due to the progression of the nuclear family and declining birthrate), (4) problems with schools (e.g., failure to establish education that emphasizes individuality, which is more suitable for a mature modernized society), (5) children's life experiences (e.g., lack of nature experiences and friendships), and (6) the impact of the development of information technology (e.g., decrease in human contact due to increased contact with information media devices).

6. The Tame-Juku program began accepting hikikomori children in 1978 (Kudō 1997, 236).

7. Therefore, Kudō could justify opening the door of the room of a hikikomori person from the outside for the sake of achieving "independence" for him, when he judges that "this child can never go out by himself" (Kudō 1997, 68–85).

8. *Retreat neurosis* is a type of neurosis proposed by Japanese psychiatrist Yomishi Kasahara in the 1970s (cf. Kasahara 1988). According to psychiatrist Naoji Kondō, it was initially assumed to be a psychopathology for which the Japanese had a high affinity, but since the diagnostic manual DSM-III, published by the American Psychiatric Association in 1980, included the diagnoses of "avoidant personality disorder" and "avoidant disorder," "it became known that these problems were not unique to Japan. In addition, . . . the cases of apathy and hikikomori were absorbed into these diagnostic categories" (Kondō 1997, 1159).

9. Psychiatrist Naoji Kondō, who contributed "The Present State of Non-Schizophrenic Hikikomori" (Kondō 1997) to this special issue, already described the "non-schizophrenic withdrawal syndrome" at the World Congress of Psychiatry in 1996. Most of the psychiatrists who contributed to the special issue of the *Japanese*

Journal of Clinical Psychiatry shared this context of "non-schizophrenic hikikomori." A volume, *Adolescent Hikikomori: Psychosocial Background, Pathology, and Therapeutic Assistance* (Kanō and Kondō 2000) used "non-schizophrenic hikikomori" and "non-psychotic hikikomori" interchangeably (Kanō and Kondō 2000, 7).

10. The Japanese word *Shakaiteki* is an adjective which corresponds to "social" in English. Saitō wrote that he used the term *Shakaiteki Hikikomori* as a literal translation of the English phrase "social withdrawal," which signifies a symptom appearing in various mental disorders. *Shakaiteki Hikikomori* means a withdrawal from all social relationships other than one's own family (Saitō [1998] 2013: 18). He uses *Shakaiteki Hikikomori* and *Hikikomori* interchangeably (Saitō [1998] 2013, 10).

11. In another article, Saitō explains the term "social participation" as "the state of being in school, working, or having intimate relationships outside the family" (Saitō 2002, 22).

12. The social structural reason why this state of hikikomori is continuous and stable is because they are forced to be included by their families in a situation where there is no other support for their life security, as described in chapter 3.

13. Although Saitō said, "At present, I have no intention of developing such an argument of what should be done" (Saitō 2002, 70–71), his basic stance on the necessity of therapeutic intervention seems not to have changed, saying, "Based on my personal experience, it is true that most hikikomori cases require therapeutic assistance" (Saitō 2012, 196). In the English edition of *Shakaiteki Hikikomori*, though, he added the following cautious reservation: "I do not, however, think that treatment should be carried out through coercion. We all know stories of people being held by force in psychiatric institutions—such forceful methods are not the best way to treat a patient in withdrawal" (Saitō 2013, 99).

14. This comment appeared only in the postscript of the original Japanese version.

15. The three incidents were the murder of an elementary school student in Kyoto in December 1999, the confinement of a girl in Niigata in February 2000, and the Saga bus hijacking in May 2000. For details of these incidents and incident reports, see Shiokura ([2000] 2003, 184–190) and Horiguchi (2012).

16. The Headquarters for the Promotion of Youth Development (*Seishōnen Ikusei Suishin Honbu*) was abolished on April 1, 2010, and the Headquarters for the Promotion of Children and Youth Development (*Kodomo Wakamono Ikusei Shien Suishin Honbu*) was established in its place in accordance with the Act for the Promotion of Support for the Development of Children and Youth enacted in the same month.

17. Regarding the process of introducing the concept of NEET into Japanese policy discussion, see Toivonen (2012).

18. See Honda (2006, 57–59) and Ishikawa (2006; 2007, 65–67) for more details on the joining of hikikomori support groups to NEET support measures. Yōsaku Satō of the NPO *Bunka Gakushū Kyōdō Nettowāku*, which was commissioned to run the Youth Independence School project, stated that more than half of the organizations running the Youth Independence School were organizations that supported hikikomori cases (Satō 2005). Nōki Futagami, who supported school non-attendance and hikikomori cases from the mid-1990s, wrote that "the existence

of NEETs has been in the spotlight," and that "hikikomori is positioned as a part of NEETs" (Futagami [2005] 2009, 25–27).

19. Article 4 of this outline, "Basic Direction of Measures for Youth," has a new section on "measures against hikikomori" states: "in order to deal with the problem of hikikomori, mental health welfare centers, public health centers, municipal health centers, and child guidance centers will provide consultation and support" (Headquarters for the Promotion of Youth Development 2008, 26).

20. The KHJ lobbied vigorously for the Act. See, for example, *Tabidachi* (the official newsletter of the KHJ), No. 51 (issued on July 5, 2009) and No. 54 (issued on January 10, 2010).

21. Article 15 of Chapter 3, "Support by Relevant Organizations," calls for "consultation, advice, and guidance," "medical treatment and recuperation," "improvement of the living environment," and "support for education and employment" by those who "engage in affairs related to education, welfare, health, medical care, correction, rehabilitation, employment, and other fields related to the support of children and youth development."

22. This guideline refers to a report that suggests around 10% of school non-attendance cases would be hikikomori in their 20s. It also mentioned that there must be a sizeable amount of hikikomori cases among NEETs.

23. The study by Kondō et al. was conducted based on the DSM-IV-TR (Diagnostic and Statistical Manual of Mental Disorders, Fourth Edition, published by the American Psychiatric Association), and 148 of the 184 hikikomori cases had enough detailed information to make psychiatric diagnoses (Kondō et al. 2010, 70). Only one case hadn't any psychiatric diagnosis among the 148 cases. He divided the diagnoses regarding hikikomori cases into three main groups: Group 1 included those with a primary diagnosis of schizophrenia, mood disorder, or anxiety disorder. Group 2 included those with a primary developmental disorder diagnosis such as pervasive developmental disorder or mental retardation. Finally, group 3 included those with a primary diagnosis of personality disorder, adjustment disorder, or somatoform disorder. The 147 hikikomori cases were categorized into one of these three groups, and the number of cases in each group was roughly one-third (Kondō et al. 2010).

24. The survey targets and main results are as follows. The survey was conducted in February 2009 and randomly sampled 5,000 cases between the ages of 15 and 39 nationwide. The total number of valid responses was 3,287 (65.7%). A total of 59 cases met the definition of the hikikomori group, which accounted for 1.79% of the total number of valid responses. This report calculates the hikikomori cases as follows. According to a national population estimate in 2007, the population aged 15–39 is 38,800,000. The estimated number of hikikomori cases is 38,800,000 × 1.79% = 696,000. The basic parameters are as follows: The ratio of males to females in the hikikomori group is 66.1% (39 males) and 33.9% (20 females), and the age distribution is approximately 54% for those up to 29 years old and 46% for those 30–39 years old.

25. This policy outline notes that "youth" covers post-adolescents up to the age of 40 in some policies (Headquarters for the Promotion of Support for the Development of Children and Youth 2010).

26. The following five principles are listed in this policy outline: (1) respect for the best interests of children and youth, (2) children and youth are partners in life with adults, (3) support for children and youth to establish themselves and become active members of society, (4) comprehensive support tailored to the conditions of each child and youth in a multilayered manner throughout society, and (5) reviewing adults in society (Headquarters for the Promotion of Support for the Development of Children and Youth 2010). These principles were new compared to the previous Policy Outline for Youth Development. These outstanding features of the new policy outline must be related with the fact that it was issued under not the conservative LDP but the Democratic Party of Japan administration.

27. See, for example, *Tabidachi* (the official newsletter of the KHJ), No. 44 (issued on May 3, 2008) and No. 46 (issued on September 14, 2008). As of April 1, 2021, 79 centers have been established.

28. Furthermore, a part headed "Support for children and youth who are NEET, hikikomori, or school non-attendance" states the measures for them as: (1) networking "various organizations such as education, welfare, health, medical care, correction, rehabilitation, and employment, which should provide support according to their developmental stages by utilizing their expertise;" (2) providing "necessary consultation, advice, and guidance;" (3) "establishing community councils for supporting children and youth;" and (4) providing "training to develop capable persons who provide support, e.g., on-site support (outreach)." This policy outline also requires local governments to establish a "community council for supporting children and youth."

29. As discussed in chapter 3, some researchers had already pointed out that many NEETs come from economically disadvantaged families (Socio-Economic Productivity Center 2007; Miyamoto 2015a).

30. The principles of the previous policy outline were deleted, which included: (1) respect for the best interests of children and youth, (2) children and youth are partners in life with adults, (3) support for children and youth to establish themselves and become active members of society, (4) comprehensive support tailored to the conditions of each child and youth in a multilayered manner throughout society, and (5) reviewing adults in society (Headquarters for Promoting Support for Children and Youth Development 2016).

31. Community social worker Reiko Katsube coined this word in 2016 (Katsube 2016; cf. *Asahi Shinbun*, December 30, 2017, morning edition).

32. Hikikomori UX conference (*Hikikomori UX Kaigi*), a general incorporated association of those who have experienced hikikomori, also issued a statement on May 31, 2021, which warned against media reports that linked hikikomori or the 80 50 problem with the criminal cases soon after the crime reports (Hikikomori UX Kaigi 2019).

33. Tamaki Saitō's definition of Hikikomori (Saitō [1998] 2013; see Chapter 3), which focused on the state of "not participating in society" itself, has been effective in terms of intersecting the two contexts of mental health and social independence. This is because mental health experts can work on "social participation" (*Shakai Sanka*) by focusing on individual behavior and psychology, while non-medical support

professionals also treat it in the context of social independence. Thus, the concept of "social participation" is a platform that allows different contexts, from mental health to employment support, to join in together and practices, while causing confusion in discussions in terms of mixing these contexts.

34. There are attempts to provide new employment support beyond the limitations of the support that sets the goal of full-time employment, in a form of employment called "intermediate employment," which creates an intermediate stage between full-time employment and welfare employment (Tsutsui, Sakurai, and Honda 2014). However, it is not yet prevalent in hikikomori support, and it is still uncertain whether this job support can change the postwar model of life security. Intermediate work needs not only wages but also social benefits to support the lives of diverse people who have difficulty to keep working in the current labor market system.

35. Roger Goodman (1998) insightfully explains the function of the system of voluntary welfare commissioners (*Minseiiin seido*) and the Japanese style of welfare society theory in Japanese social security system and how the theory was proposed based on the perception of the "Western" societies.

36. Based on the medicalization theory, Ogino examines the relationship between hikikomori and psychiatry using the concept of the sick role, with particular attention to the situation of hikikomori support. The sick role exempts the subject from the normal role and can lift the blame and shame for not working or attending school. The role also makes it possible to use the medical insurance system. On the other hand, however, the sick role is not always favorable. Ogino points out four important disadvantages (Ogino 2008b, 223–227): (1) the existence of stigma associated with mental illness and mental disorders; (2) unlike physical illness, the effect of exemption by mental illness and mental disorders is vague; (3) even though psychiatric diagnosis is arbitrary, it can be the definitive representation of the person diagnosed; and (4) diagnosis can have complicated effects on the course of symptoms (e.g., the diagnosis causes those around the person to abandon their efforts to understand the person, and in response to their attitudes, the person sees himself or herself as sick and establishes a fixed identity as a sick person).

Chapter 5

On the Difficulty of Participation

From Theoretical and Empirical
Considerations of the Situated Self

FOCUSING ON THE SITUATION RATHER THAN
THE PSYCHOLOGY OF HIKIKOMORI SUBJECTS

This chapter considers hikikomori subjects' difficulties in participating in interactional situations with others. Why do hikikomori people avoid interactions with others? What difficulty do they experience in participating in such situations? There are many approaches to these questions, and one of the most convincing approaches is to explore the psychology of hikikomori subjects, which emphasizes the importance of recognizing who and what hikikomori people are. The representative theory of this approach is based on E. H. Erikson's identity theory. Several studies on the hikikomori experience refer directly or indirectly to it (Kuramoto 2002; Sakurai 2003). They take both psychology and the intersubjective relationship between one and others into account to explain the problem of self-identity that a hikikomori person experiences. The essential focus is on how hikikomori subjects experience a lack of recognition of who and what they are by their significant others.

This chapter will point out the successes and limitations of Erikson's psychological approach and then propose a different approach: Erving Goffman's sociological theory of the situation and the situated self, which focuses on the structure of the situation. In the following sections, I will first examine how Erikson's theory analyzes the difficulties in participation of hikikomori subjects and clarify the limitation of this approach. Then I will show how Goffman's situational approach, which focuses on the situation and the actors who are defined by the situation rather than individual psychology, can clarify the difficulties in participation for hikikomori subjects.

DIFFICULTIES IN PARTICIPATION
FROM THE PERSPECTIVE OF ERIKSON'S
THEORY OF SELF-IDENTITY

Narratives and Interpretation Regarding Lack of Recognition

Why do hikikomori subjects find it difficult to participate in situations involving other people? Psychologists and counselors who try to help hikikomori people have often interpreted this difficulty as a lack of recognition of who and what they are by others (Tanaka 2001; Hironaka 2003). Many hikikomori subjects also describe their personal experiences of lack of recognition from others. As quoted in chapter 1, hikikomori subject Kazuki Ueyama said, "In the world, only *my* voice is isolated," and "I am definitively alone" (Ueyama 2001, 142). For Ueyama, society alienates him and provides no recognition of his self (see chapter 1). Another hikikomori person describes his experience just before he went into hikikomori status as follows: "There was no one who would listen to how I felt. Everyone just imposed their own values and the values of general society, and I didn't feel like saying anything. At least at that time, there were only such people as had those values, and I didn't have anything else I wanted to do, so I had to push myself hard to go to school" (Hagiwara 2001, 205). No one acknowledged what he felt, so he "didn't feel like saying anything" to those around him. Finally, his patience reached its limit, and he started avoiding interactions with others.

Another hikikomori person said that recognition was vital for her to get out of hikikomori status: "Thanks to my husband, I experienced being loved just as I am. He gave me a feeling of stability that I had never had from my parents. He never judges me or ignores me. He treats me as a human being" (Shiokura [1999] 2002, 165). According to her, the experience of being accepted "as I am" by her significant other was essential to recovering her inner stability and her ability to interact with others.

Mutuality as a Requisite for Self-Identity

As seen above, hikikomori people often talk about their experiences of rejection instead of acceptance, neglect instead of recognition. Psychologists and counselors have found a lack of acceptance and recognition in the hikikomori subjects' psychological background as an explanation for their avoidance of human relationships.

The theoretical framework most relevant to this psychological experience is E. H. Erikson's self-identity theory. Erikson argues that it is crucial for a youth's identity formation that he or she "be responded to and be given a function and status as a person," and this response means that he or she is "recognized" (Erikson 1968, 156). A fundamental lack of recognition would cause people to form a basic distrust of others and themselves, leading to an identity crisis (Erikson 1968, 254).

Before discussing identity crisis, however, let us first review the essential perspective of identity formation. Erikson argued as follows:

> Identity formation . . . begins where the usefulness of identification ends. It arises from the selective repudiation and mutual assimilation of childhood identifications and their absorption in a new configuration, which, in turn, is dependent on the process by which a society (often through subsocieties) identifies the young individual, recognizing him as somebody who had to become the way he is and who, being the way he is, is taken for granted. (Erikson 1968, 159)

Erikson points out two things here. First, he distinguishes between *identification* and *identity formation*. Although identification is a passive process in which one unconsciously internalizes role expectations from others, identity formation is an active self-formation in which one consciously selects and integrates identifications. Secondly, identity formation is underpinned by a reciprocal relationship between the ego and the other. Self-identity is supported by others, who recognize the self as he or she who does or does not respond to expectations from others. This recognition from significant others is essential to form the self-identity of the person.

The reciprocal relationship between the self-image of oneself and the self-image for others, which he calls "mutuality," constitutes self-identity. Erikson states that

> The young person, in order to experience wholeness [as a sense of coherent inner identity], must feel a progressive continuity between that which he has come to be during the long years of childhood and that which he promises to become in the anticipated future; between that he conceives himself to be and that which he perceives others to see in him and to expect of him. (Erikson 1968, 87)[1]

Self-identity is a sense of "sameness" between one's self-image and that of others, as well as a sense of "continuity" from one's past self to one's anticipated future self. The latter signifies the temporal perspective of the self. Thus, senses of sameness and continuity are both essential for identity formation. Accordingly, identity formation requires sameness between the self-image which one conceives and the self-image which one perceives others conceive.[2] The mutuality of self-image also has a temporal aspect, which is the continuity of the past self and the participated future self.

Hikikomori Experience as an Identity Crisis

When society does not recognize who and what the person is and who and what the person will be, one cannot assume the mutuality that underpins identity formation. An *identity crisis* occurs in such a situation. An identity crisis is an experience of discrepancy between the self-images. This experience causes the feeling of isolation and lack of recognition in Erikson's sense. In an identity crisis, one feels anxious about exposing oneself to others because one cannot assume the mutuality of self-image, and the opacity of the mutuality of self-image leads to anxiety, fear, and confusion.

To a certain extent, identity crises can explain the withdrawal of hikikomori subjects from face-to-face interaction. Withdrawal is avoidance of others because one feels the anxiety, fear, and confusion of an identity crisis. Sociologist Tatsushi Ogino describes this difficulty of hikikomori people from a perspective compatible with Erikson's identity theory as follows:

> It is difficult to feel the validity of one's sense of self in this world with a certain degree of certainty without experiencing the expression and acceptance of one's preferences, however seemingly trivial they may be. . . . If we thoroughly lack such experiences, it will be extremely difficult for us to embrace a somewhat affirmable image of ourselves that allows us to expose ourselves to and engage with others. (Ogino 2008a, 152)

An identity crisis also explains prolonged withdrawal behavior. Withdrawal behavior from interpersonal interactions does not solve an identity crisis. Instead, a withdrawn state can worsen the discontinuity in self-image because people in withdrawal might be blamed for their withdrawn state without any recognition of who and what they are (see chapter 1). Thus, withdrawal behavior as a coping strategy for an identity crisis leads people to a dilemma: the more they avoid interactions and withdraw deeply, the less that significant others recognize them in a way which secures the mutuality of self-images.[3]

Journalist Yutaka Shiokura describes this vicious circle of hikikomori, focusing on two aspects: the vicious circle of psychology and the vicious circle of interaction. First, withdrawal behavior leads the person to become more isolated, and a certain period of withdrawal and isolation in turn deprives them of confidence to take steps back into society. Thus, the trauma of lack of recognition creates a new trauma via withdrawal. This process is the vicious psychological circle. Second, the more people withdraw, the more their parents feel anxious and blame their withdrawn children harshly. This situation distances people in withdrawal more and more from interactions with their parents. This process is a vicious circle of interaction. These dual vicious circles prevent hikikomori people from escaping their withdrawn state, even when they want to (Shiokura [2000] 2003, 221–229). This convincing analysis of the persistence of withdrawal is also consistent with Erikson's identity crisis theory, which focuses on the intersubjective recognition of the person.

DIFFICULTIES IN PARTICIPATION FROM THE PERSPECTIVE OF GOFFMAN'S THEORY OF INTERACTION

The Need to Focus on the Logic of the Situation

Although Erickson's self-identity theory provides a convincing explanation for both the psychology of the subject and interaction mechanism that deprives the recognition of a person, it seems necessary to go one step further into an analysis of the situation in order to understand hikikomori people's difficulty of participating in a situation with others. Empirically speaking, hikikomori people do not avoid all situations involving others. Many hikikomori subjects can and do participate in some situations, such as joining a self-help group, meeting a few friends, or going to a convenience store or a library (Ishikawa 2003b).

This empirical fact contradicts a theoretical assumption of the identity theory, which focuses on the fundamental identity crisis, because the identity crisis cannot explain these participations in particular situations. Therefore, we need a theoretical framework that can explain the empirical fact that hikikomori subjects can and do participate in certain situations in which other people are involved. To explore this point, Alfred Schutz's view on participating in a situation gives us an important clue. He says:

> Except in the pure We-relation of consociates, we can never grasp the individual uniqueness of our fellow-man in his unique biographical situation. In the constructs of common-sense thinking the Other appears at best as a partial self, and he enters even the pure We-relation merely with a part of his personality. . . . My constructing the Other as a partial self, as the performer of typical roles or functions, has a corollary in the process of self-typification which takes place if I enter into interaction with him. I am not involved in such a relationship with my total personality but merely with certain layers of it. In defining the role of the Other I am assuming a role myself. In typifying the Other's behavior I am typifying my own, which is interrelated with his, transforming myself into a passenger, consumer, taxpayer, reader, bystander, etc. (Schutz [1953] 1962, 18–19)

While sharing these insights with Schutz, Erving Goffman considered a situation in which people coexisted as an autonomous system and developed his argument of the situation which exceeds individual actors. Goffman's work, *Frame Analysis: Reflections on the Organization of Experience* (Goffman 1974), focuses on the frame of a situation that "organize[s] participants' experience" within it.

A *frame* is the context of a situation, the mutual awareness of the definition of the situation shared by participants (Scheff 2005). People acquire knowledge of the shared definition of a situation as socially approved, taken for granted, prior to participating in the situation. People also individually perceive "what is going on here" and they can form mutually shared knowledge of this awareness, or the definition of the situation, in the course of interaction. Goffman considers the shared definition of the situation as a frame, and explores the constitution of a self in relation to this frame.

The Situated Self as a Derivative of a Situation

According to Goffman, not only a role but also a person in a situation is a resource that the participants utilize to maintain the orderliness of a situation. Regarding the relationship between a role and the person who plays it, Goffman says:

> The individual comes to doings as someone of particular biographical identity even while he appears in the trappings of a particular social role. The manner in which the role is performed will allow for some "expression" of personal identity, of matters that can be attributed to something that is more embracing and enduring than the current role performance and even the role itself, something, in short, that is characteristic not of the role but of the person—his personality, his perduring moral character, his animal nature, and so forth. . . . There is a person and role. But the relationship answers to the interactive system—to the frame—in which the role is performed and the self of the performer is glimpsed. Self, then, is not an entity half-concealed behind events, but a changeable formula for managing oneself during them. (Goffman 1974, 573)

To distinguish between role and person, Goffman proposes a "person-role formula" (Goffman 1974, 269), which treats participants in a situation on a continuum of role and person; participants recognize each other as combinations of role and person, where the latter is irreducible to a role. A person is a player who plays a role in the situation, and the player is, so to say, a meta-role, "the role of interactant" (Goffman [1957] 1967, 116).[4]

Goffman emphasizes that the situation generates the person-role of participants. He writes that "the sense of the person beyond the role, is, or certainly can be, a product of what becomes locally available," and "[a] sense of the person can be generated locally" (Goffman 1974, 298). Thus, we can produce a personality of participants based on the performances of participants in a current situation. Individuals in a situation pick up on each participant's role performances as available cues for recognizing their person and together create an integrated entity—a "person-role." Thus, as sociologist Tadafumi Kimura points out, cognition about the person of a participant and his or her biography is "a cognitive product derived from roles which are utilized as resources in each situation" (Kimura 2015, 67). Typifying participants according to the person-role formula is achieved by picking up the attributes, capacities, and information of the actor available according to the shared definition of the situation.

Goffman says: "Whatever a participant 'really is,' is not the issue. . . . What is important is the sense he provides them through his dealings with them of what sort of person he is behind the role he is in" (Goffman 1974, 298). In Goffman's view, participants construct the person performing a role in a situation. In this sense, the self is derived from the situation.

Participation and the Person-Role Formula

In his article "Embarrassment and Social Organization" (Goffman [1956] 1967), Goffman points out that "things go well or badly because of what is perceived about the social identities of those present," and then goes on to say:

> During interaction the individual is expected to possess certain attributes, capacities, and information which, taken together, fit together into a self that is at once coherently unified and appropriate for the occasion. Through the expressive implications of his stream of conduct, through mere participation itself, the individual effectively projects this acceptable self into the interaction, although he may not be aware of it, and others may not be aware of having so interpreted his conduct. At the same time he must accept and honor the selves projected by the other participants. (Goffman [1956] 1967, 105)

The "acceptable self" is a combination of person and role appropriate in a certain situation. It is not a substance beyond each situation, but what the individual projects into the situation and what other participants interpretively construct by gathering "his stream of conduct" according to the definition of the situation.

This perspective suggests that a change in context could resolve the difficulty of participation without any change in participants. For example, consider the testimony of hikikomori subject Kazuki Ueyama: a natural disaster changed the context (shared definition of the situation) and thereby made it easier for him to participate. He experienced the Great Hanshin-Awaji Earthquake of 1995 in his hometown in Kobe while still in a state of withdrawal. He wrote about his experience as follows:

> The fact that I could not buy a single rice ball even if I had a 10,000-yen bill [approximately 87 US dollars] made me feel unusually free. My daily life was broken, and I was on the verge of death, but there was nothing to bind me. When I breathed, I felt that I was breathing through my own lungs. It's not the senseless breathing that is constrained by norms. The situation of "turning on the faucet, but no water comes out" made the norms disappear. I was thrown out with others into the middle of nowhere. I was "socially active," as a matter of course. (Ueyama 2006)

In the immediate aftermath of the earthquake, a different definition of the situation arose, and Ueyama could engage in social activities as a matter of course.

In the context of everyday life, some particular person-role formula is dominant—for example, an adult male stranger in a residential area during the daytime on a weekday can be considered as a suspicious person.[5] However, in a disaster situation, the everyday life definition of the situation is lifted and no longer relevant—a different context arises. Under the context of an extraordinary situation, the same adult male can be treated as a normal person, for example, as someone who helps remove debris. This case is a clear example of how the frame and the corresponding typification of oneself and others a person-role formula—are rendered. Such a transformation of the definition of the situation orders a person-role combination differently, which can make participation easier.

Regarding the recovery of the context of everyday life as time passed after the earthquake, Ueyama writes:

> This "freedom" and impressive "attitude to cooperate with each other" disappeared like a receding tide as the lifelines were restored. Once again, there was the uncomfortable relationship among residents in which "I don't want to get involved." Once again, the oppressive circuitry of "everyday life" started up. . . . .. The monetary economy has begun. Once again, that "suffocation" has begun. (Ueyama 2001, 77)

As the lifelines that support everyday life recovered, the context at the time of the earthquake gradually changed. As a person-role formula appropriate to the context of everyday life returned, Ueyama felt difficulty participating in the situation again. An adult male individual in a situation of a daytime residential area on a weekday cannot be considered a properly behaving person anymore. What makes participation more challenging here is not the change of the participant but the change in the context and the person-role formula according to that context.

Achieving Proper Person-Role in Mr. B's Case

Although Ueyama's case shows a change in the context can either promote or hinder participation, Goffman also pointed out that "through the expressive implications of his stream of conduct, through mere participation itself, the individual effectively projects this acceptable self into the interaction" (Goffman [1956] 1967, 105). This suggests that even when the context does not change, self-presentations or performances *can* change: participants can be proper to the context by presenting themselves skillfully. For example, a hikikomori male may always wear a suit when he goes out to convenience stores as a part of his performance to maintain the appearance of a normal person which is proper to the definition of the situation.[6]

Let me illustrate this point in detail with the case of a hikikomori subject, Mr. B. After experiencing hikikomori status for about two years in his mid-20s, he joined a support group for hikikomori cases and acquired new personal relationships. The following is a narrative of a situation in which his friend invited him to a dinner with people he had never met before:

> When we all had dinner together, six or seven of us, I went over and [my friend] said, "This is B. He is a hikikomori." Without any pretense, out of nowhere [my friend said this]. I would say, "Oh, it's nice to meet you." Then he would say, "Oh, I'd like to introduce you all to B, a hikikomori." He's that kind of guy. He doesn't understand [me], in a good way. I've always said that it's good to have a person who doesn't understand you. That's how I was really trained. So, at first, . . . I was awkward. I tried patching up like, "Ah, no . . . ," but then everyone would lose interest. "What's wrong with him? He is awkward." So, I learned from that and made my speech compact, so it's a self-presentation. In a few dozen seconds, I would compactly say, "Ah, well, there was a time when I was like that." So, I've been trained at a few dinner parties. I've become able to say, "Well, there was a time like that." If I didn't do that, [the situation] wouldn't move forward. You see, when everyone comes to eat and to talk, I shouldn't take up too much of their time with my incomprehensible personal stories. I understand that. So, I say, "Yes, yes, I am it [a hikikomori]."

He describes how he felt embarrassed in the situation yet became able to perform appropriately to the situation. His friend all of a sudden introduced him to other participants as a "hikikomori." At first, Mr. B was embarrassed by that. He had no idea what kind of performance was proper to the situation, and it was also difficult for him to distinguish between what was relevant to him and what was relevant to the context of the situation. However, he gradually discovered performances proper to the context. This insight is summed up in the words: "When everyone comes to eat and to talk, I shouldn't take up too much of their time with my incomprehensible personal stories." He learned how to present himself in a "compact" way that is proper to the context in which "everyone comes to eat and to talk."

This episode suggests that embarrassment can offer an opportunity to learn what is relevant in a situation as well as how to perform and present oneself properly to the definition of a situation. Mr. B realized others' reactions to him ("What's wrong with him? He's awkward.") and learned how to achieve the common perception of a person-role proper to the situation.

THE SITUATED SELF AND SELF-IDENTITY

Imagining a Person as a Virtual Focus

In a person-role formula, participants treat each other according to the definition of the situation. Thus, there seems to be no room for a whole person to appear in the situation in Erikson's sense of self-identity. The wholeness of the individual that transcends actual circumstances has a serious theoretical discrepancy with Goffman's conception of the situated self, which is embedded and produced in a shared definition of a situation.

However, some hikikomori subjects have narrated their experiences under the framework of the self-identity theory. Mr. B also refers to his self-presentation as a hikikomori person in the dinner situation as follows: "To some extent, I reduce myself, but even if I reduce myself, I realize that it isn't shocking, and it doesn't undermine my spirit. It also can make others laugh." Here, he recognizes that a situated self is a self which is relevant to the definition of the situation, and that it is a partial self. At the same time, he mentions another aspect of his self as his "spirit" in contradistinction to the reduced self-presentation. This "spirit," unlike the reduced self in situations, seems to be a self that is detached from any situation. Thus, a sense of self-identity that goes beyond the situated self still has some importance. How can we reconcile these two approaches to the self?

A person-role formula is applicable to the recognition of self for oneself in a situation, though we have mainly discussed the recognition of self for other participants. A participant experiences performing a role and being treated as an appropriate person in some situation. In addition to this recognition of person connected to the role performed in a certain situation, he or she gradually forms an image of his- or herself who can participate and be treated as a proper person in various situations. This self-image is an image of the person that transcends each and every situation, yet is still rooted in the situated self. Although this process is seemingly similar to identity formation in Erikson's theory, this person is not a substantial self, but rather an imaginary self that transcends and is underpinned by a particular person-role combination in each situation.

The person that one conceives transcends a situation is a *virtual focus* for one's ego. A "virtual" focus suggests a point from which the rays of light seem to emanate; it is a perceived light source that does not actually exist. By assuming the imaginary person as a virtual focus for the ego, participants can interpret each situated self as a fragment of this person. The person cannot exist in the actual situation but works as a reference point to the situated self in each situation.

Although the person as the virtual focus is an imaginary image of oneself conceived by collecting situated selves, once the person as the virtual focus is formed, it will begin to function for the ego as if the imaginary person is the precondition for participation, for participants themselves are under the illusion that this self as the virtual focus is a prerequisite for participation in situations. Thus, there is a circular relationship between the situated self and the person as a virtual focus. The accumulation of the situated self supports the virtual focus, and the virtual focus supports each participation, although this process often goes unnoticed: it is taken for granted that there exists a positive circular relationship between one's person and one's situated selves. Mr. B, for instance, became able to perform his situated self skillfully, and that did not undermine his imaginary self as his "spirit," because of this positive circular relationship.

Between the Situated Self and the Self-Identity

If the person as the virtual focus is formed only as a by-product of accumulation of participation in situations, then it would be a reckless attempt to acquire such a self before participating in concrete situations. Furthermore, as Mr. B suggested, it is considered inappropriate to be concerned with the self-image of a whole person, for that would be irrelevant to the definition of the situation. If a participant sticks to his or her whole person, which is not relevant to the situation, then he or she can stray away from spontaneous involvement in the situation. As Goffman observed, "to be self-conscious or other-conscious is in itself an offense against involvement obligations" (Goffman [1957] 1967, 125). The offense against the "involvement obligation" causes other participants to consider the individual as "a faulty person," as Goffman says: "A person who chronically makes himself or others uneasy in conversation and perpetually kills encounters is a faulty interactant; he is likely to have such a baleful effect upon the social life around him that he may just as well be called a faulty person" (Goffman [1957] 1967, 135). Goffman pointed out that the offense against involvement obligation even endangers the order of the situation: "Unless the interactants regain their proper involvement, the illusion of reality will be shattered, the minute social system that is brought into being with each encounter will be disorganized, and the participants will feel unruled, unreal, and anomic" (Goffman [1957] 1967, 135). Thus, "the role of interactant is something he will be obliged to maintain" (Goffman [1957] 1967, 135).

However, unlike Mr. B, who could finally achieve a robust circulation between his situated self and his imaginary person (his "spirit"), some hikikomori subjects experience serious distress by concentrating on properly performing their situated selves. Yuki Sawada, who researched female hikikomori subjects, mentioned that they suffer from trying to achieve a proper situated self in each situation:

> Although all four subjects [interviewees] were able to "play" the situated self which is required by others in each situation, they all had an Eriksonian person as their "true self," which is inseparable from difficulties and distress. Thus, it was a common outline that they are tired from and torn between the awareness of falsity of hiding those difficulties and presenting the situated self, and as a result, they withdraw from interaction situations. Presenting a situated self is a primary form to protect their "true self" inseparable from difficulties, but others do not recognize their attitudes, and they become exhausted and withdraw as a secondary form of protecting themselves. . . . They referred to the situated self as the "fake self" or the "decorated self" and contrasted it with the "true self"—their whole self-identity—that was fraught with difficulties and could not do things as other people do. In other words, their self is a duality of "fake" and "true." (Sawada 2021, 11)

While recognizing the definition of the situation and presenting themselves as proper situated selves, they cannot secure the imaginary person as a self-image that can participate in various situations. To be precise: the more they focus on properly performing their situated selves, the more they feel exhausted by the distance between their "fake self" and their "true self." They recognize that the situated self never overlaps with their "true self." How can the polarity of the situated self and the imagined self as a virtual focus form a positive loop in these cases? If concentrating on both the situated and integrated selves could interfere with a positive circulation between them, how can hikikomori subjects resolve the difficulty of participation in interaction situations?

If both over-attachment to self-identity and over-involvement in the situated self impede the positive feedback between the person as a virtual focus and the situated self, one strategy available to hikikomori people is to strike a balance between the two. On the one hand, that is to accumulate embarrassing participations as a situated self (as Mr. B did),[7] and on the other hand, to look for situations in which they can participate with a proper person-role formula without feeling excessive stress. Other hikikomori subjects have also talked about such experiences. Mr. C said, "There are more books on bicycle racing than in most bookstores [in my room]," and he would go to bicycle races, even if he had to force himself a little to do so. Ms. D liked live music so much that she would go to live concerts at night. Even among hikikomori subjects, there are many different situations in which they consider they can and want to participate.

This discussion of the situated self suggests that hikikomori people do not need to train themselves to participate in situations. What they need to do is not to make an effort to change themselves in order to participate, but rather to think calmly about the quality of situations where one would want and might be able to participate without excessive stress or a huge burden to "fake" themselves. If using the hikikomori category seems to facilitate participation in the situation, then use it; otherwise, avoid its use. For example, one hikikomori subject never introduced himself as hikikomori when he participated in a gathering for his hobby. On the other hand, he introduced himself as a hikikomori when he participated in a meeting to talk about hikikomori experience. This selective use is a good strategy for hikikomori people to participate in situations with ease.

Practical Implications for Hikikomori Support People

The proper person-role in a situation is correspondent to the shared definition of the situation as a mutual awareness, and the way it is applied is often self-evident. Thus, it is not something a single participant can control at will. So then, if other participants try to mitigate the hikikomori subject's difficulty in participation, what is required is not to try to change the subject but to reflect on how the current definition of a situation makes it difficult for him/her to participate in the situation and to create a situation that facilitates participation.

A specific context creates difficulties in participation. One hikikomori subject said that he always felt uncomfortable in the family setting because of the constant focus on him as a problematic person. When he watched a TV program in the living room with his father, and there was a story about a young athlete's success, his father sighed and said, "Why don't you make an effort like him?" In the family setting, the dominant definition of the situation determined him as a hikikomori son deserving of contempt rather than respect. This situation made him feel uncomfortable participating in conversations in the family settings. He found it easier to participate in family conversations as a listener—for example, sitting quietly at the table while his parents enjoyed talking about a recent domestic trip. In that situation, he was not treated as a problematic person, although his role as a son remained the same. Ueyama's post-earthquake episode also suggests that a situation in which other participants recognized him as a normal person made his participation more manageable. Even in Mr. B's case, his friend who introduced him as a hikikomori without any special care indicated that it is "normal" to experience a state of withdrawal, and this treatment may have cultivated a context which made it easier for Mr. B to participate in the situation.

Thus, a context where any individual is treated with respect as a person is a minimum condition to foster hikikomori people's participation. People from different backgrounds (such as those who are bullied, unemployed, disabled, or sexual minorities) know that there are situations where they will not be treated with respect, and this expectation will discourage them from participating in those situations. The challenge is how to cultivate a shared definition of the situation where diverse types of "person" can play a "role" with respect.

Support professionals may recognize a hikikomori individual as a problematic person by identifying themselves as support professionals. With reflection on this unintended consequence, some hikikomori support professionals suggest that it is important for the support person to have a relationship with hikikomori subjects on an equal footing, in which hikikomori subjects join in the assessment and have a dialogue about what their needs are and what sorts of support they want, rather than the support person unilaterally deciding the goals and methods of support (Yamamoto 2013). This is a way to create a context in which people are treated as equal participants with respect.

In addition, the very definition of the situation as a place for providing support defines the target of support (hikikomori subjects) as inferior individuals, because the concept of "support" implies a participant has a problem that requires support. This kind of situation can reinforce the difficulty hikikomori people face when participating in situations. Regarding this point, Yasuhiko Maruyama proposes a *non-supporting* relationship with hikikomori people in the family situation (Maruyama 2014). Maruyama argues that relating to a hikikomori subject as a normal family member (such as asking for help with household chores or having a dog and taking care of it together), rather than treating him or her specifically as a hikikomori, is important to improve the relationship. These treatments are trials to change the definition of the situation, which do not assume that hikikomori subjects need to be supported.

Given how this chapter has focused on hikikomori subjects who can and do go out in some situations, one might now ask about severe hikikomori cases, where subjects cannot even leave their own rooms. Regardless, the argument in this chapter remains the same. From the perspective of the situated self, interactions through a bedroom door are also situations of interaction, and it is necessary to reflect on the definition of the situation: how it makes participation in the situation stressful, and how to change not the individual but the situation by focusing on the definition of the situation and the person-role formula assumed in the situation.

CONCLUSION

This chapter has discussed self-identity and the situated self and argued that achieving not self-identity but a positive circulation between situated selves and an imaginary self is essential. This is valid not only for hikikomori subjects but also for those who have never experienced hikikomori status. As Goffman puts it: "The present situation defines the public appearance which we hide ourselves behind. In exactly the same way, the present situation gives us a place to reveal our true nature, a way to reveal our true nature. Culture itself dictates what kind of entities we must believe ourselves to be in order to have something to reveal in this way" (Goffman 1974, 573–574).

This chapter suggested that where various person-roles can appear with respect, the difficulty of participation in the situation can be mitigated. Following the discussion in this chapter, supporting hikikomori subjects requires people to make more than an effort to change them; it requires people to make an effort to focus on changing the situation that prevents hikikomori subjects from participating. It raises the question of how we can cultivate a context in which hikikomori people are not treated as inferior and in need of correction, but as human beings with their own unique struggles.

NOTES

1. Erickson distinguishes between "wholeness" and "totality" of self-identity (Erikson 1968, 80–82). Wholeness is a state in which diverse elements are integrated. In contrast, totality is a state of uniformity in which diverse elements are truncated. A healthy self-identity is associated with a sense of wholeness, not totality.

2. Erikson confirms that "the human environment is social, the *outerworld of the ego* is made up of the egos of others significant to it" (Erikson 1968, 219; italics in the original text). How the egos of others conceive oneself is not comprehensible.

Thus, one's recognition of the mutuality of one's self-image is nothing but what the ego itself perceives.

3. Ishikawa (2007, Chap. 3) offers the insight that the withdrawal behavior is prolonged by (1) the degree of anonymity in a situation and (2) the degree to which they are made aware of their stigma in a situation. Her explanation also focuses on the situation, and she concludes that withdrawal behavior is a means to protect themselves. Her analysis is important in respect that she focuses on the characteristics of the situation. However, she doesn't explore either the relationship between the self-identity and the situated self or how the situation creates the difficulty in participations. This chapter examines these issues.

4. To recognize a participant as a person means to treat him/her as a full interactant who plays multiple roles in a situation. Goffman (1963, Chap. 6) mentions various situations where participants are not recognized as persons, and calls such participants "non-persons." They are not treated by others with respect as social objects but as physical objects. As examples, Goffman refers to the treatment of slaves: a "very young lady lacing her stays with the most perfect composure before a negro footman," and "a Virginian gentleman" who has "a negro girl sleep in the same chamber with himself and his wife" (Goffman 1959, 95). In both cases, the slave man and girl are treated more like physical objects than persons. Non-personhood is, of course, not an inherent property of black people, but a product of the shared definition of the situation (the frame).

5. In contemporary Japanese society, wherein the male-breadwinner model is still assumed, adult males are expected to be working full time, so only elderly people and female housewives are expected to be present in residential areas during the daytime on weekdays.

6. This example is from a case in a NHK program on the hikikomori problem (NHK Kurōzu Appu Gendai 2011). He is in his 40s and has been in a hikikomori state since he failed to get a job when he graduated from university.

7. Goffman discusses participating in situations with ease: "It should be nearly as evident that almost every activity that any individual easily performs now was at some time for him something that required anxious mobilization of effort. To walk, to cross a road, to utter a complete sentence, to wear long pants, to tie one's own shoes, to add a column of figures—all these routines that allow the individual unthinking, competent performance were attained through an acquisition process whose early stages were negotiated in a cold sweat" (Goffman 1971, 248). The positive circulation between the situated and integrated selves may be formed after accumulating such participations.

Chapter 6

Time Perspective in the Hikikomori Experience

TIME IN THE NARRATIVES OF HIKIKOMORI EXPERIENCES

Hikikomori subjects have a problem with time perspective. This chapter will examine how they come to regain a time perspective for the future by considering their hikikomori experiences from storytelling. Ryōko Ishikawa, a sociological researcher of hikikomori, refers to the importance for hikikomori people of "being able to imagine oneself continuing to live in whatever form" by citing the "sense of the future" of A. Giddens (Ishikawa 2007, 216–217; cf. Giddens 1984, 62). She argues that a "sense of the future" is formed by addressing "existential problems," for example, "how we should live" by "digging deep inside" (Ishikawa 2007, 218–229). This chapter also examines Ishikawa's argument regarding these existential problems.

There are indeed characteristic narratives of hikikomori subjects regarding their time perspectives. These narratives describe "the lack of time flow" or "the lack of movement of time." Although Ishikawa focused on the "sense of 'future,'" she did not analyze the time perspective in the hikikomori experience in detail.[1] Therefore, this chapter takes up the perspective of hikikomori subjects and analyzes it from narrative theory to clarify how the sense of "lack of time flow" arises, and then this chapter examines how they regain a time perspective. This perspective is deeply related to the ambivalence discussed in chapter 1 and the social structure of life security discussed in chapter 3.

NARRATIVE THEORY OF TIME

Time has present, past, and future phases. These phases are interrelated: the future is ahead of the present, and the past is behind the present. However, hikikomori subjects often describe that the relationship between the present and the future is disconnected during their hikikomori condition. For example, Sekimizu (2016) refers to a response from a hikikomori subject to the question, "When you were in hikikomori condition, did you think you would stay at home with your parents for a long time?" "'For a long time' wasn't what I thought. I was not thinking about the future. I couldn't think about it, and I didn't understand it. The right now at the moment was everything. . . . The present was everything. I didn't have the ability to think about the future." Kazuki Ueyama, a hikikomori subject, recalls the time when he began working part-time as a tutor at a prep school and bought his first schedule book at the age of 31: "For me, who had been living only in the suffocating sequence of 'now, now, now,' this [schedule book] was unfathomable. Once you've written it down and made a promise, you have to be bound by it" (Ueyama 2001, 104).

Both subjects look back at their time perspective in their hikikomori experience as a succession of "presents" without any discernible "future." How should we interpret the narratives of their time perspective during the hikikomori experience?

Another hikikomori subject said that she felt that she was just living because she could not die, and she withdrew utterly in order to push herself into a corner to have "the courage to commit suicide" (Tanabe 2001, 27). She expresses her "feeling of being alive because I cannot die" as follows: "The ordinary person sees the way ahead that will lead to the future, such as his life after five years or ten years later, doesn't he? I didn't see things this way. When I looked behind, there was a road on which I had walked, but when I looked ahead, the road ended in front of me, and I could see nothing but darkness" (Tanabe 2000, 28). This account gives us a clue how to interpret the time perspective of hikikomori subjects and understand their lack of future perspective. The "ordinary" person sees a future life that connects their present with their future, even with vague vision. Without this time perspective, they cannot live a life in a time flow—that is, they do not regard the moments of their life as having a clear progression from past to present to future.

Some hikikomori people say that the future is not there. It's not just that they have difficulty seeing the future clearly, but they cannot see the future at all. They express a more intense feeling that there is no future to which the present can be connected. Ms. D makes this point even more explicit:

I was on the edge of an abyss, and there was only darkness in front of me. It was like a black hole, and I didn't know which way to go, not even one step. The path was cut off. . . . I was just standing still. It was not like I was looking back and regretting the past. I was looking ahead, but at a black hole. At that time, there was really no information about credit-based high schools or the university entrance qualification examination, and I had no options at all when I quit [high school].

Ms. D was in her second year of high school in the mid-1980s and was unable to go to school after the "Golden Week" holidays[2] due to her deteriorating health, and this narrative is her description of her feelings when she finally dropped out of high school. Why did Ms. D lose her sense of the future by dropping out of high school?

Dropping out of high school at that time was, how to say it, like the ultimate in something that should never happen, and it really shut the future off. At that time, the only people who dropped out were delinquents. There were a lot of delinquents who dropped out of school, but that was for a different reason. No, neither my family nor anyone thought that would happen in my life.

For Ms. D, who attended a preparatory school, dropping out of high school was an event that neither her family nor she herself had expected. Ms. D describes her feelings at that time as follows: "Even after quitting school, my physical condition did not improve. I was mentally trapped and felt like my life was over. It was the only way I knew: to go to university and get a job. So I felt that my future was gone" (Tanabe 2000, 199).

Ms. D's narratives suggest two points. First, the time perspective is structured as a story that leads from now to the future and gives direction to one's life. The storyline Ms. D told involves going to university and getting a job. By arranging life events in a time series from past to present to future, we make up a story of life. This story gives direction to the present life. The story must have a future to which the present points, and a past is from which the present has come, that points to the present. As David Epston and Michael White, narrative therapists, say: a story is "a unit of meaning that provides a frame for lived experience" and enables "persons to link aspects of their experience through the dimension of time" (Epston and White 1992, 97).[3]

Second, the story that creates the time perspective becomes disorganized when the present is dislocated from the storyline. In this case, the reality in which the person lives becomes nothing but a sequence of disoriented present moments. Such disorientation results from the absence of the future to which the present moment points, which Ms. D expressed. The medical sociologist Arthur W. Frank describes the situation in which the storyline connecting present and future is demolished as a "narrative wreck," borrowing a phrase from Ronald Dworkin (Frank 1995, 54; cf. Dworkin 1993, 211).

Frank considers a sense of temporality to be "the central resource that any storyteller depends on." As an empirical study, he discusses the narrative wreckage that occurs in the experience of illness. The experience of illness wrecks the narrative "because its present is not what the past was supposed to lead up to, and the future is scarcely thinkable" (Frank 1995, 55).

Narrative wreckage must be seen not as the story's disappearance, but as a "disjunction" between the story and the reality in which a person lives. He says: "The stories we have in place never fit the reality, and sometimes this disjunction can be worse than having no story at all" (Frank 1995, 55). The experience of illness is not part of the storyline that organized experience in the past, present, and future sequence. For this reason, the experience of illness renders the story that organized the person's experience dysfunctional. The person is unable to find the future to which his/her present leads.

Then, what kind of story is wrecked by the hikikomori experience? Ms. D's narrative, quoted above, has a typical storyline: "It was the only way I knew: to go to university and get a job; so I felt that my future was gone." Other hikikomori subjects mention the wreckage of the "from school to work" storyline. After the summer break of his first year of high school, Mr. B, who experienced hikikomori in the early 1990s, was suddenly ignored by all his classmates without knowing why. He continued to attend high school and describes his feelings at that time as follows:

> Of course, I didn't have the option of not going to school. There were no alternative schools. If I dropped out, I would be out. I don't know how I survived. I thought, "For now, until I reach the second grade [of high school]." I thought, "That's a long time. What will happen to me? But I can't quit [high school]. I can't quit because of my parents." Some students dropped out of our high school, and I wondered what they were going to do. I wondered what they would do now. I would have become a school non-attender. . . . Twenty years ago, it was still *Tōkōkyohi* [school refusal]. The word "*Futōkō*" [school non-attendance] was not widely used, and the image [of school refusal] was that of a complete dropout. I think that's what everyone in their 30s [i.e., the same generation] thought. They thought they couldn't drop out [of high school].

Sekimizu (2016) discussed another hikikomori subject, born in the late 1980s and who went to school in the late 1990s and later, whose narrative also contains the storyline of "from school to work." In response to the question, "Did you feel that you did not want to go to school?" she responded:

> I wanted to go to school, but it was hard. I remember my mother and father telling me many times in elementary school and junior high school that I didn't have to go to school. However, for some reason, I was stuck in the mindset that I have to go because everyone else is going. I also wanted to see my friends. I

was convinced that I have to go, and if I don't go [to school], I won't be able to work properly, I guess.

Although the causes of the narrative wreckage of hikikomori subjects are diverse, the common storyline hikikomori subjects share is the path "from school to work." As discussed in chapter 3, after the period of rapid economic growth from the 1950s to the early 1970s, the normative life course was to graduate from high school or go to university and then get a stable job immediately after graduation. This storyline was taken for granted by most of the Japanese population under the developmentalist social policy. Thus, the life course "from school to work" became the dominant expectation.

THE WAY OUT OF THE NARRATIVE WRECKAGE

The Teller of the Restitution Narrative

According to Frank, the solution to narrative wreckage also lies in telling stories (Frank 1995, 55). So how do hikikomori subjects find a future to which the present leads and thereby reclaim the story of their lives?

One way is to change the present, which has deviated from the storyline, and reposition it closer to the original storyline. In the case of the hikikomori experience, this means going back to the "from school to work" storyline. This approach is often the first one that hikikomori subjects try. Most of them make efforts to return to the dominant storyline. In so doing, they become teller of what Frank calls a "restitution narrative."[4]

The restitution narrative has the following basic storyline: "Yesterday I was healthy, today I'm sick, but tomorrow I'll be healthy again." The core expectation of this narrative type is the return of the person to the *status quo ante*, the status of "I'm fine!" (Frank 1995, 90). With respect to the hikikomori experience, a typical restitution narrative would have the form: "I used to be in hikikomori condition, but I have recovered from it and returned to society."

The restitution narrative sets the status of going to school or work as the goal of the storyline—in other words, reintegration, but it ignores the question of why such status is the goal.[5] The tellers of the restitution narrative never question the legitimacy of the goal. Behind the restitution narrative "lies the modernist expectation that for every suffering there is a remedy" (Frank 1995, 80). Not only hikikomori subjects but also their families hope for them to become tellers of restitution narratives. Returning to the "from school to work" storyline is very often the shared hope of the hikikomori person, their families, and support professionals.

Nevertheless, it is not easy for a hikikomori subject to become a teller of the restitution narrative. For most subjects in the midst of a withdrawn state, the story of their lives has lost its plot and has fallen into chaos. When everyone expects the hikikomori person to reintegrate into society and hopefully be a teller of the restitution narrative, they unintentionally ignore the experience of narrative wreckage in the present.

What hikikomori subjects really need is to have a witness to their current narrative, which has no storyline: the chaos narrative (Frank 1995, 97–98). Frank argues as follows:

> The need to honor chaos stories is both moral and clinical. Until the chaos narrative can be honored, the world in all its possibilities is being denied. To deny a chaos story is to deny the person telling this story, and people who are being denied cannot be cared for. . . . Those living chaotic stories certainly need help, but the immediate impulse of most would-be helpers is first to drag the teller out of this story, that dragging called some version of "therapy." Getting out of chaos is to be desired, but people can only be helped out when those who care are first willing to become witnesses to the story. (Frank 1995, 109–110)

Honoring the chaos narrative means simply listening to the chaos experienced by the person in the wreckage, without imposing on them the restitution narrative, or any narrative at all.

Some hikikomori people encounter "witnesses" to the chaotic story, who accompany the narrative wreck and the process of trial and error of retelling the story. For example, Naomi Hayashi, the author of *I Didn't Want to Be a Hikikomori* (Hayashi 2003), is one such hikikomori subject. She could not go to junior high school and later experienced the hikikomori condition. After that, however, she entered and graduated from university, went to and completed graduate school in the United States, and then worked in Tokyo. Her autobiography seems to follow a typical restitution narrative, which shows her process of recovery: "I used to be hikikomori, but now I'm fine."

The retelling of her story was not accomplished by her alone. She wrote about a young man she met at a church, who listened to her chaotic narrative as a witness: "At first, I didn't even know what I wanted to say, but little by little, I began to be able to talk. In the beginning, I think, all that came out of my mouth were negative words. 'I am afraid,' 'I am lonely,' 'I don't know what is going on,' and 'I need help . . .' However, he accompanied me, who couldn't say anything positive" (Hayashi 2003, 93–94). After that, she could meet with various people who honored her chaotic stories: her first best friend, a piano teacher she considered her mentor, and a doctor she could trust. Through these encounters, she was able to tell her story. The doctor she met "kept repeating [to her] that 'you were not bad and that even if your parents did not accept you, you could live'" (Hayashi 2003, 109). With the support of these people, she came to accept the wreckage of her narrative.

She mentioned another reason for her "smooth reintegration into society," which was "encountering senior people who could be role models" for her life. She wrote:

> One of the scariest things about being in a school non-attendance or hikikomori status is that you lose the vision of your own life and the image of what kind of person you want to be. When you meet someone who can show you concrete examples of how people can live and how people can think, you will be able to see the image little by little. (Hayashi 2003, 123)

She gradually gained witnesses to her narrative wreckage, which helped her establish a new connection from her present to her future, in a way bringing her back to the "from school to work" storyline. Role models showed her a future with which her present situation could connect. She seems to be a typical teller of the restitution narrative. In fact, in her book, she writes: "Of all my friends, I was the one who was able to return to society most smoothly" (Hayashi 2003, 122), and "I was able to leave school normally, work normally, talk to my friends normally, and fall in love normally" (Hayashi 2003, 191).

However, in the same book, she also wrote, "I still have psychological scars that I cannot forget, even if I want to forget" and "When I remember my past and become aware of my trauma, I feel as if my social life, which has finally begun to move, will break down, and I will even lose myself again" (Hayashi 2003, 162). Thus, even after becoming a storyteller of the restitution narrative, she continues to be mired in chaos without a plot.[6]

What is vital in achieving the restitution narrative is to discount experiences that do not fit into the restitution plot. The tellers of the restitution narrative have to believe in "the modernist expectation that for every suffering there is a remedy" (Frank 1995, 80), and never question the goal of the *status quo ante* as reintegration into society.

Skepticism about the Restitution Narrative

Not all hikikomori subjects tell restitution narratives. There are cases in which they cannot find a way out of the narrative wreckage even after changing the course of their present to return to the original storyline. By examining such cases, we can clarify the limitations of the restitution narrative.

Again, Kazuki Ueyama, a hikikomori subject, is one such case. After dropping out of high school for the second time, he passed the entrance exam and entered a university, but he could not escape from the feeling of "groundlessness" (Ueyama 2001, 51), as if he was in the middle of nowhere. He describes that he felt anxious wherever he was and whatever he was doing, and thus absolutely groundless (Ueyama 2001, 58). Where did his sense of groundlessness come from, which persisted even after he became a university student? Why did Ueyama not become a teller of the restitution narrative, even though he recovered the present according to the "from school to work" storyline?

Before he experienced the hikikomori condition, Ueyama believed that the only possible life course was going to school and getting a stable job. He wrote: "The image of becoming an adult was obsessively installed in my mind as a 'single rail track,' and I believed that to keep going on that rail track as long as possible was the only approved way for 'adults.' Dropping out meant death" (Ueyama 2001, 40). For him, the typical "from school to work" storyline was oppressive. He wrote the following episode about his junior high school days in the early 1980s:

> There was a time when my father did not come home for a month. When I asked my mother why, she said, "Don't be silly. He comes home every day." To my surprise, he came home around one o'clock after I went to bed and got up around five o'clock, before I woke up, to go to work. . . . I was truly horrified. I thought, I must go this far to be allowed to "become an adult," and this is what it means to "enter society." (Ueyama 2001, 41)[7]

Ueyama felt that the original storyline itself was deadly oppressive. He also wrote that "learning and working meant nothing but 'slavery to the time axis' [in a society]," and described how the concept of a "single rail track" from school to work was tormenting him (Ueyama 2002).

Ueyama continued to desperately play his role in the "from school to work" storyline; but he became exhausted, and as a result fell off the "single rail track." Seen in this light, the reason he could not get away from the narrative wreck even after entering university is apparent. For him, the original storyline itself was a source of despair. Even so, he could not imagine any other storyline for his life, because, as he wrote, "dropping out meant death." He tried to somehow put his present back into the original storyline, but the future to which the present should lead remained invisible.

Ueyama's case raises doubts about restitution narratives in the hikikomori experience, which hikikomori subjects themselves, their families, and support professionals often take for granted. As a result, those hikikomori subjects who cannot become tellers of the restitution narrative may need to create alternative stories to rebuild from their narrative wreckage.

Creating Alternative Stories

The narratives of two hikikomori subjects, Mr. F and Ms. D, suggest constructing a life story different from the restitution narrative. In the late 1970s, Mr. F was unable to attend high school and experienced the hikikomori condition. He repeated the first year of high school four times, and from the fifth attempt he attended school for three years without a break, taking seven years to graduate from high school. Before the fourth repeat of the first year, he blamed his parents for four days and four nights because he was so upset about the possibility that he would be expelled from high school.

> On the fourth night, I started thinking, "I don't mind quitting [high school]" for the first time. Before that, I kept thinking I really didn't want to quit. . . . My mind changed; what matters is not graduation from high school but my life. It was a Copernican revolution for me. When I realized that my life was more important than school, it was as if a fog had lifted. It was like a light shining into a spring in the forest. All the resentment and obsession with my parents flowed away into the water of the fountain. The next day, I was able to go to school naturally, whereas I had forced myself to go before that.

After graduating from high school, Mr. F went on to college, hoping to become a teacher. However, after graduating from university, he fell into a state of withdrawal again. It took seven years for him to recover from his withdrawn state. He described the change in his mindset before recovering from his second hikikomori episode as follows:

> [At that time] I couldn't find a job, and I couldn't participate in society. I thought that I was useless to this society and that the day would come when I would die, and no one would notice it. I felt like the world of death was right beside me. Then one day, without any trigger, I thought, "That's fine." I began to think, "Just dying and becoming earth without anyone caring about me. Since the human being is also an animal, such a way of dying is fine. Since I am that level of a person, let my life and death take their course, like a wild animal."

For Mr. F, the future to which the present could lead was not school or work but death as a wild animal. Such a death was the future to which he could believe the present would lead. Death is not necessarily something to be avoided for Mr.F, unlike now death is typically conceptualized. Finding death as a wild animal meant finding life as a wild animal. He was able to reclaim the future by telling a "wild animal life" storyline instead of the "from school to work" storyline. Mr. F also said, "I am living without the premise that I am a human being." The story of the life that Mr. F reconstructed is not the restitution narrative but the story of just living and dying as a wild animal.

Ms. D's narrative is also very different from the restitution narrative. After quitting high school, she passed the University Entrance Qualification Examination and entered a university.[8] However, after about two months she quit university because it became too hard to force herself to keep attending. Ms. D talked about the 20 years since she stopped going to high school as follows: "I was trying to survive in the [underground] world below the world where everyone else lived. I felt like I was living in a different world."

Referring to Mr. F's narrative of his getting out of school non-attendance, Ms. D said she saw an image similar to Mr. F's when she escaped from her withdrawn state: "The image of water flowing from a spring into a river." She continued: "I thought that was the source of my life. When I saw that image, I thought, 'I have come back to life.' I also have the awareness that I was born just to live and die. One day I will surely die, and I just think I will live until that time." Ms. D thought of her life like water flowing from a spring, the flow of which rises in her present, toward her death. She also created an alternative plot of her life instead of returning to the dominant "from school to work" storyline.

Mr. F's story of "life as a wild animal" and Ms. D's story of being "born just to live and die" are both expressions of alternative stories at odds with the dominant life story of "from school to work," which presupposes a sequence of social roles based on one's belonging to social groups or organizations. Recognition of one's own death relativizes the narrative of "from school to work." Thinking about death reminds storytellers that it is not someone else but they themselves who die and that what matters is their own lives. This recognition of oneself as a unique being contrasts with the impersonal time perspective of the dominant storyline.

Mr. F expressed this view of life as the "life of wild animal," and argued, "They say there are many paths in life, but in reality, there is only one path." He wrote:

> If I were to compare life to a path, I would say, "There is only one path for each person, and each person walks on his or her path from birth to death." As long as there is only one path for each person, there is no way for a person to go off-course (deviate) or take a detour. Everyone is walking on a single path. The path has flat parts, bumpy parts, steep parts full of stones and weeds, and tunnels with no visible exit. Therefore, as long as they walk, they all have to pass through a steep path at times. (Mr. F's e-mail newsletter, April 23, 2003)

No matter what kind of rough path it is, to live a life is to keep walking a path, and a person will continue to walk that path until death. This motif is common in both Mr. F's and Ms. D's alternative stories. In their alternative stories, and there is no such thing as "going off the path." Whatever the path is, they are on the right track.[9]

RECONSIDERING THE PROCESS OF RETELLING

The Dominant Story and Unique Subjectivity

For both Mr. F and Ms. D, the awareness of death was an opportunity to recognize the uniqueness of their own subjectivity, which is irreplaceable, unlike social roles. This awareness encouraged them to liberate themselves from the dominant story, the "from school to work" life course. This dominant story is not rooted in the uniqueness of the subject, but in a life story as a series of social roles. As the previous chapter explained, Japanese society has formed a situation wherein private companies and families hold tremendous responsibility for people's life security during the period of rapid economic growth from the 1950s to the 1970s and the subsequent completion of the Japanese style of welfare society. During these periods, the "from school to work" life course is legitimated as a part of an "already given" social world.[10]

Hikikomori subjects deviate from this legitimated life course. Hikikomori subjects cannot tell their stories through anonymized, impersonal narratives. They are forced to discover novel storyline that would give words to their individual experiences. Becoming aware of death offers an opportunity to relativize the anonymous, impersonal life story and take on an alternative life story rooted in the uniqueness of the subject.

Telling "Our" Hikikomori Stories

How, then, are the collective nature of the hikikomori category and the uniqueness of each hikikomori experience reconciled by subjects' narratives? Ishikawa (2007, 117) refers to Peter L. Burger and Thomas Luckmann's following discussion: "For instance, I have a quarrel with my mother-in-law. This concrete and subjectively unique experience is typified linguistically under the category of 'mother-in-law trouble'" and "In this way, my biographical experiences are ongoingly subsumed under general orders of meaning that are both objectively and subjectively real" (Berger and Luckmann 1966, 53–54). Do the narratives of hikikomori subjects achieve a collective character via the category of hikikomori? Do they establish the first-person plural, "our" story of the hikikomori experience?

On this point, Ms. D clearly states that "I cannot speak for [the hikikomori experience of others] because individual situations and circumstances are different. What I consider important is that the person him/herself speaks in his/her own words" (Field Notes, March 25, 2012). For Ms. D, being a hikikomori subject does not entail that she can speak for the collective meanings of "our" hikikomori experience. Therefore, Ms. D elects not to speak for other hikikomori experiencers.

However, her assertion that each hikikomori subject has a unique story that others cannot share does not mean that the narrative of hikikomori experience cannot be a collective "our" story. Rather, Ms. D is arguing that the first-person plural, "our" story of hikikomori experience always requires recognizing unique aspects of each hikikomori experience. "Our" hikikomori story does not have unified storyline, but we each experience a unique struggle to confront both society and ourselves.

Interactive-Practical Process of Retelling

This life-story retelling process should not be thought of as being accomplished only through the storytellers' self-reflection. As mentioned at the beginning of this chapter, based on Giddens' concept of "futural" sense (Giddens 1984, 62), which is a sense of routine based on "ontological security," Ishikawa targeted a "mental work" to "put one's experiences and feelings into words" and to answer "existential questions" like "How do I live?" or "What do I work for?" or "Is my existence worthwhile?" (Ishikawa 2007, 222 and 230). Ishikawa emphasizes how this kind of self-reflection and verbalization serves as a recovery process for hikikomori subjects.

It would be misleading to focus solely on the self-reflection associated with solitary cognitive action. Ms. D discusses how she encountered diverse people whom she met in the hikikomori group, as well as her doctor, who kept telling to her, "I have hope for you." She said:

> Those two things [involvement in the hikikomori group and dialogue with the doctor] were significant. I think it would have been hard for me if I had only one of them alone. I could grow my personal roots, and I could make connections with others and expand my world and convince myself, "I am not alone, and there are many ways of life." Doing both things at the same time was very significant for me.

Both narrative processes—to grow personal roots and to make connections with others—proceeded simultaneously and with the support of both relationships with the hikikomori group and the psychiatrist.

Naomi Hayashi, a teller of the restitution narrative, also recovered her life story little by little thanks to the people who witnessed her narrative wreckage. Mr. C underlined the importance of people who just listen to his story without any advice (see chapter 1). Even Mr. F, who discovered his life as a wild animal, said that it was essential for him that he encountered in a study meeting for school social workers those who shared his will to change not the individual, but society. Those encounters were of huge significance in motivating him to return to social activity.

Underscoring the solitary self-reflection may avert our eyes from the isolation of hikikomori subjects, wherein they lack witnesses of the chaos narrative and are forced to focus on solitary cognitive work. As Ms. D said, hikikomori people require the processes of growing personal roots and making connections with others, and both are supported by witnesses to the narratives of hikikomori subjects.[11]

In addition, Giddens positioned "existential problems," for example, trust in others and a sense of integrated self-identity, as problems at the level of practical consciousness rather than discursive consciousness. Thus, solitary self-reflection at the level of discursive consciousness alone neither answers nor solves those existential problems at the level of practical consciousness. Hikikomori subjects could give words to their chaotic experiences through dialogues with themselves and with witnesses to their narrative wreckage.

CONCLUSION

Hikikomori subjects experience narrative wreckage when they deviate from the dominant story of the normal life course "from school to work." Then, they struggle to accept the present and to discover the future to which their present could connect, with the support of witnesses to their narrative wreckage. This retelling process is not limited to the tellers of alternative stories, but is also true for the tellers of the restitution narrative who aim to return to the dominant storyline. The tellers of the restitution narrative are also trying to accept their present, which deviates from the dominant story.

This process of retelling is also a process of alleviating the ambivalence in hikikomori experience, but it is not a unidirectional process toward social participation. As the alternative story clearly shows, the process of alleviating the ambivalence is also a process of affirming a self who lives at a distance from the majority society. In other words, it is a process of finding one's own way of engaging with society between the two vectors of participating in society and distancing oneself from society.

There might be a question regarding the usage of the word "story" to interpret the narratives of hikikomori people: does "story" imply the fictitious character of their narratives? I used the term "story" because the stories of hikikomori lives are created, retold, and changed and that their stories are always in the process of generation. However, the process of hikikomori subjects shows that they cannot create their life story at will. They must find a life story that they truly believe in, in their biographically determined situations. They seek to find a life story they can believe in as they encounter witnesses to the lives they lead.

NOTES

1. Kaneko (2006) discusses the difference between time management in hikikomori support facilities and time management in the "society" outside the facilities. In contrast, this chapter focuses on the narrative of time in the hikikomori experience. The field of psychology has accumulated research on time perspective (cf. Ishikawa 2013; Okuda 2008, 2013). These psychological studies have conducted quantitative and qualitative analyses that have provided interesting insights such as a relationship between evaluation of the past and future perspective (Ishikawa 2014). However, those psychological studies do not refer to narrative theory.

2. The "Golden Week" is a week-long holiday during early May in Japan.

3. David Carr, citing Edmund Husserl, argues that there are three aspects of temporality in human experience: the temporality of passive experience, the temporality of action, and the temporality of the narrative structure of the self/life. The first is the temporality of future grasping. The first temporality is found in the melodic experience of sound through grasping the future and grasping the past, the second temporality is found in the fact that action is a series of bodily actions located in a certain context and is not divisible, and the third temporality is found in the narrative structure that creates a continuity of action and experience (Carr 1986). These three aspects, as Carr points out, are interrelated and cannot be treated independently. However, this chapter focuses mainly on the third temporality.

4. The restitution narrative is one of the three basic types of narrative that Arthur Frank posits. The other two are the "chaos narrative," which has no narrative order, and the "quest narrative," in which the teller takes on suffering as his/her quest.

5. Frank points out that the restitution narrative prefers a future which brings recovery and is disinterested in the genesis of the suffering (Frank 1995, 88–89).

6. She cannot completely eliminate the chaos narrative from her life story. In the Translator's Afterword of the Japanese translation of Frank's book, Tomoyuki Suzuki, wrote that "the chaos narrative" is a basic component of the story (Suzuki 2002, 282–283).

7. This harsh working style is an example of the "*Kaisha Ningen*" [company-centered man] discussed in chapter 3.

8. By passing this examination, one can have the qualification to take the university entrance exams without graduating from high school. Its name was changed to the "high school equivalency examination" in 2005.

9. However, for Mr. F and Ms. D the chaos narrative remains, even in their alternative stories. Mr. F said, "I don't know if I am glad that I experienced hikikomori, but I think it was a life of living in uncertainty, and that is what my life is about." Ms. D also says, "I can't say that I am glad that I experienced hikikomori because I lost so much, but my life has become richer because I experienced hikikomori" (Field Notes, November 16, 2008).

10. Alfred Schutz and Thomas Luckmann write: the "individual experiences the social world which is already given to him and objectified in the relative-natural view, as a scale of subjective probabilities related to him, as an ordering of duties,

possibilities, and goals attainable with ease or with difficulty" (Schutz and Luckmann 1973, 95).

11. The processes "to grow my personal roots" and "to make connections with others" can be gleaned from the ambivalence hikikomori subjects experience, which chapter 1 of this book discussed. The former overlaps with the process to recognize and be faithful to one's own nature and the latter is to meet the expectations of others.

Conclusion

Japanese Society in the Light of the Hikikomori Experience

THE HIKIKOMORI EXPERIENCE AND CONFORMISM

Conformism and Its Social Background

This final chapter will reflect on what has been discussed and draw a conclusion. It is clear from what has been discussed so far that hikikomori subjects do not voluntarily choose to be excluded from social participation. Rather, most of them want to participate in society, especially school and work, according to the expected life course as defined by the majority. However, at some point, they face an inability to conform to the majority life course any further (chapters 1 and 6).

In a hikikomori condition, people become surrounded by other people's questions, like "Why can't you keep going to school or work?" or "Why won't you move out of your parents' house?" They feel guilty and anxious that they cannot live up to the expectations of others and consequently they deny themselves. This feeling of guilt and anxiety occurs because most hikikomori subjects desire, at least initially, to conform to the majority life course at the level of discursive consciousness.

This conformity, which is shared between hikikomori people and others who ask the rhetorical questions (chapter 1), is a realistic adaptation under the *Japanese-style of welfare society* policy. This policy assigns the responsibility for securing people's living to private corporations and families and has intentionally reinforced conformity since the late 1970s. Under this private-sector-oriented life security system, hikikomori subjects are forced into severe conflicts with family members (especially parents) and are desperate for employment. Parents, too, are forced to exert intense pressure on their jobless children to work when their families must provide life security for jobless family members, which deepens the conflict between parents and children and makes their relationship more difficult.[1]

The cases of Ueyama and Katsuyama, who were born in nuclear families in the early 1970s, notably show a normative orientation coincident with the majority track under this policy idea. Under this principle of the policy, they were thrown into a competitive school system to get stable job status in stable corporations and experienced severe conflicts with their parents after they deviated from "from school to work" story line. They took the majority life course as the only possible "rail track" for living, according to which deviation from the track is fatal. For example, Ueyama confessed his assumption that coming off the track "from school to work" meant death. Also, Ms. D mentioned that she felt as if she lived in an "underground world" after she dropped out (chapter 6). In this way, some part of the mental suffering of hikikomori subjects is certainly a product of the life course model under the social security policy in postwar Japanese society, which imposes on families and private companies the maximum responsibility to provide life security for citizens.

As discussed in chapter 6, some hikikomori people relativize the absolute superiority of the majority path and thus detach themselves from blind conformism through the recognition of their own nature. Then they can confront the self-addressed questions to find their own styles of social participation. People like Katsuyama fight proactively against conformism by giving up the majority way of life. Other hikikomori subjects, like Ueyama and Mr. B, do not give up the majority path but try to find a means of survival. In each case, this process of affirming their own way of social participation requires relationships with others who see and hear and thereby affirm their suffering and ambivalence.

The Ambivalence and Nature of Hikikomori Subjects

Hikikomori hope to go back to the majority track at the discursive consciousness level, but they have more complex or ambivalent experiences at the practical level (chapters 1 and 6). They often deny their maladjusted selves, yet they cannot change their hikikomori condition because they feel ambivalent about the nature of their selves at the level of practical consciousness, which is sometimes invisible. Thus, there is an inconsistency between the discursive and the practical consciousness. This gap makes it difficult for other people to understand the hikikomori experience. Adopting the term "hikikomori" is a way for them to express their ambivalence (chapters 1 and 2).

Chapter 1 discussed how hikikomori subjects experience ambivalence about their own nature. They "wish" to meet the expectations of others and, at the same time, they "want" to respect their own nature. The latter sometimes goes unrecognized even by themselves at the level of discursive consciousness. Hikikomori subjects struggle to meet the expectations of those who want them to conform to the majority track. However, the majority track entails a progression "from school to work," and what full-time male worker or housewife status requires makes it difficult for some to follow this majority track.

The hikikomori subject's own nature is often experienced just as an "inability" to conform to the expectations of others, and it is difficult for hikikomori subjects to accept their nature. The expectation to conform to the majority track is too coarse-grained an image of social participation, because it ignores the unique nature of each individual. The expected social participation, which is molded according to the Japanese style of welfare society policy, leads hikikomori subjects to conceive of their nature as an "inability" that need to be corrected. Hikikomori people are not permitted to search for self-acceptance of their natures in diverse situations or to explore their relationships with others. Rather, they are forced to despair. The suffering of hikikomori subjects comes not only from conformism but also an assimilationism which only allows for specific kinds of social participation in line with the "from school to work" track. The next section discusses this issue.

The hikikomori subject's own nature is not clearly grasped from the beginning, even by hikikomori subjects themselves. Just as the self-as-virtual-focus is constructed through participation in various situations (chapter 5), the nature of the self is not apparent from the beginning for hikikomori people themselves, thus it must be grasped through concrete participations and concrete reactions from others in concrete situations.[2] A recognition of the nature of the self that ignores its situation-constructing aspect would be useless for hikikomori subjects themselves. It is the relationship between the self and society, not the self alone or society alone, that must be explored in order to understand the hikikomori experience.

THE HIKIKOMORI PROBLEM AND ASSIMILATIONISM

Japanese Life Security System and Assimilationism

It is necessary to think about the difficulties that hikikomori subjects experience from the other angle, by focusing on the majority of people who do not experience the hikikomori condition. From this perspective, the conformism of hikikomori subjects is not a problem of their personal attitude, but a problem of the assimilationist character of Japanese society, which impels them to their conformist efforts.

Assimilationism is the idea of integrating the distinct natures of different people—their different thoughts, values, and ways of living—to the majority's preferred way of being.[3] This book has suggested that the assimilationism that characterizes the hikikomori condition is a product of the postwar Japanese social security system, which increased the responsibility of corporations and families for life security. The male breadwinner earns a living wage to support his family while females take hands-on care of their family members, and the welfare state tries to avoid conferring direct benefits for life security as long as possible (chapter 3).

Cultural anthropologist A. Borovoy argues that postwar Japanese society has tried to include as many people as possible in mainstream society. Therefore, the mechanisms at work in the mental health system, in schools, in families and businesses, and elsewhere seek to "warehouse" the maladjusted or otherwise marginalized people into dedicated segments of the mainstream, wherein they are expected to assimilate over time (Borovoy 2008, 564). The mainstream refers to the majority life course, and more specifically to "the spectrum of middle-class values" (Borovoy 2008, 554–555). Conformism to the mainstream is a prevalent and realistic coping strategy in Japanese society.

The Assimilationism and Pursuit of Happiness

In postwar Japanese society, people have forced themselves to conform to the majority life course, and they also force others—especially their children—to do so, too, often with the best intentions. They are assimilationists and conformists at the same time. Public support for hikikomori cases is essentially premised on this idea, which aims to set them on the "from school to work" life course (chapter 4).

Those non-hikikomori who have assimilated and conformed to what the majority defines as "normal" consider those who seek to accept and live by their minority natures to be selfish. The more they abide by the majority life course, the more harshly they may criticize a minority stance. This oppressive attitude toward the minority is a projection of the oppression they impose on themselves in order to stay on side of the majority. In postwar Japan, many people struggled to fit the mainstream conception of the modern family in order to survive, and more or less ignored or suppressed their own natures. In the case of certain types of disability, like cerebral palsy, in which a person is apparently "different" from the majority, it may be easier for the majority to accept that someone has their own style of committing to society.[4] However, regarding many hikikomori cases, the reasons for being isolated are not always easy to understand at first glance. In these cases, the assimilationist demands will not stop. People continually question why hikikomori people behave the way they do, and hikikomori people also question themselves in the same way (chapter 1).

The hikikomori experience thus raises the question of assimilation to the majority in society. The standpoint of assimilationism takes the majority as its standard, and it considers the goal of any effort to support hikikomori cases to be reintegration into mainstream society. However, hikikomori subjects reconsider and relativize the assimilationism of the majority path. From their perspective, our society consists of those who have different natures and different biographical backgrounds, which are invisible from the assimilationist standpoint.

The problem raised here concerns the dream of a society that oppresses oneself and others as little as possible and supports everyone to pursue their own happiness. The hikikomori experience and the 80 50 problem clearly show the fact that the Japanese social security system, which leaves the responsibility for life security to the family, private corporations, and now the community does not work very well. While the Japanese-style welfare society policy emphasized the Japanese labor market as a key element of life security after the late 1970s, it has noticeably lost its inclusiveness as a provider of life security since the late 1990s. In a labor market that has become increasingly exclusive, the number of people who have stable life security via the labor market has inevitably decreased. Hikikomori people can be regarded as those who have fallen into long-term joblessness supported by their parents outside the diminished labor market. As discussed in chapter 4, the concept of the *community-inclusive society (Chiiki Kyosei Shakai)* does not reflect the actual conditions of community.

Chapter 1 argued that there is a ubiquitous feeling among hikikomori subjects that they cannot and do not want to participate in society unless and until they deny their own natures. This may appear to be unforgivable selfishness to their families, because, when the family is responsible for the life security of long-term jobless people, the family and not the welfare state must play the main role of exerting paternalistic pressure toward employment.[5]

There are many arguments to the effect that hikikomori subjects are spoiled people who do not realize the harshness of society in line with the position of their parents. Psychiatrist Tamaki Saitō states that the hikikomori condition is a pathology caused by disavowing "castration" (Saitō 2013). *Castration* in this context means to recognize "through their interactions with other people that they are not all-powerful, almighty beings," in other words, it is "the act of giving up on the notion that one is almighty and powerful" (Saitō 2013, 173). He argues that the current Japanese educational system "compels students to disavow castration" (Saitō 2013, 173). Such an argument regards hikikomori subjects as immature and childish people, and it is often convincing even for hikikomori subjects themselves.

However, this book has underlined different aspects of the hikikomori phenomenon and thereby aimed to see them in a different light. First, the hikikomori problem for the family is a problem of family-dependency, which is reinforced by Japanese social security policy.[6] This problem calls for the easing of parents' financial and physical obligations to their jobless adult children, rather than their spiritual growth. Second, in terms of suffering in the hikikomori experience, hikikomori subjects search for practical options for survival in the Japanese life security system, seeking a sense of security with others whom they can trust.

CONCLUDING REMARK

This book has explored the hikikomori experience and the hikikomori problem from multiple angles. In the midst of an assimilationist social structure and in the face of difficulties finding a realistic option for living, hikikomori subjects search for their own ways to forge authentic relations with others. The hikikomori experience is characterized by suffering under such structural conditions, involving severe conflicts with parental and societal expectations. Studying how they survive isolation sheds light on an essential aspect of the relationship between individual and society, and it suggests that a stronger form of social solidarity is possible. Compared to a society that leads some people to deny their own natures by forcing them to participate in ready-made arrangements, a society that supports all people without demanding that they deny their own natures would be much healthier. I contend that the struggle of hikikomori subjects is a struggle for such a society. It is necessary to accept the hikikomori experience for what it is: not a challenge to force some people into preexisting social structures, but a challenge to foster a more inclusive society predicated on solidarity—a society that supports everyone in their pursuit of happiness.

NOTES

1. As Nicolas Tajan says, "hikikomori" is not a syndrome in psychiatry, but rather an "idiom of distress" (Tajan 2021; Nichter 2018). For parents, it is an idiom that expresses their burden of endless support duty for their jobless children, and for hikikomori subjects, it is an idiom that expresses their suffering to find their own ways to relate to society. This book has clarified the socio-structural context in which people require and use the idiom of distress of hikikomori: a life security system formed along the *Japanese-style welfare society* policy that assumes life security by corporations and families. In the absence of a new way to provide life security in response to the increasing exclusion of corporate welfare—although a new policy

idea of *community- inclusive society* has been proposed without substantial provision of life security—the distress of individuals and their families is prolonged. This situation is the basis for the widespread use of the term "hikikomori" as an idiom of distress in Japanese society.

2. It is true that the definition of a situation (the context) as a mutual awareness of the situation defines the appearance of the self, as chapter 5 discussed. However, the nature of the self is not completely reduced to the definition of the situation (the context). The appearance is, as Arendt observed, defined by the other, yet the nature of the self and their experience of it do exist and they cannot be reduced to the appearance to others. Hikikomori subjects are searching for a way to understand and accept their own natures, which often appear just as an *inability* to comply with the majority track (chapter 1).

3. As seen in colonial assimilationism, there are times when a minority forces the majority to assimilate. In other words, the term is used to refer to the assimilation of the subordinate group into the dominant group's social status hierarchy or power structure.

4. Assimilationist regimes may assign disabled people, who live in different bodies from the majority, an inferior minority position, one that is distinct from the majority path. Additionally, the majority may interpret the efforts of minority people make to rehabilitate as attempts to get closer to a majority-defined body.

5. A series of studies by Minoru Kawakita analyzes how parents experience and cope with their children's hikikomori condition (Kawakita 2003, 2004, 2005, 2006, 2008).

6. See Sekimizu (2021), which also develops this argument.

References

Aoki, Michitada, Yoshiko Sekiyama, Chūichirō Takagaki, and Bunrō Fujimoto, eds. 2015. *Hikikomoru Hito to Ayumu* [*Walking with Withdrawn People*]. Shin Nihon Shuppan-sha.

An, Juyoung, Chenweil Lin, and Toshimitsu Shinkawa. 2015. "Nikkan-tai no Kazoku-Rejīmu no Tayosei" [Diversity of Family Regimes in Japan, South Korea, and Taiwan]. In *Fukushi Rejīmu* [*Welfare Regimes*], edited by Toshimitsu Shinkawa. Minerva Shobō.

Arendt, Hannah. [1958] 1998. *The Human Condition*. The University of Chicago Press.

Aruga, Kizaemon. [1965] 2001. "Marriage and Family, Children, and Society" [*Kekkon to Ie, Kodomo, Shakai*]. In *Aruga Kizaemon Chosaku-shu IX: Ie to Oyakubun Kodomo* [*Aruga Kizaemon's Works: Family and Boss-and-his-henchmen*]. Mirai-sha.

Borovoy, Amy. 2008. "Japan's Hidden Youths: Mainstreaming the Emotionally Distressed in Japan." *Culture, Medicine, and Psychiatry* 32, no. 4: 552–576.

Cabinet Office. 2010. *Wakamono no Ishiki ni kansuru Chōsa (Hikikomori ni kansuru Jittai Chōsa)* [*Survey Report on Youth Consciousness (Fact-finding Survey on Hikikomori)*]. Accessed February 17, 2022. https://www8.cao.go.jp/youth/kenkyu/hikikomori/pdf/s2.pdf.

———. 2011. *Hikikomori Shiensha Dokuhon* [*Handbook for Hikikomori Support People*]. Accessed February 17, 2022. https://www8.cao.go.jp/youth/kenkyu/hikikomori/handbook/ua_mkj_pdf.html.

———. 2016. Wakamono no Seikatsu ni kansuru Chōsa Hōkokusho [Survey Report on Youth Living]. Accessed February 17, 2022. https://www8.cao.go.jp/youth/kenkyu/hikikomori/h27/pdf-index.html.

———. 2019a. *Seikatsu Jōkyō ni kansuru Chōsa Hōkokusho* [*Survey Report on Living Conditions*]. Accessed February 17, 2022. https://www8.cao.go.jp/youth/kenkyu/life/h30/pdf-index.html.

149

———. 2019b. *Reiwa Gannen-ban Kodomo Wakamono Hakusho* [*FY 2019 White Paper on Children and Youth*]. Accessed February 17, 2022. https://www8.cao.go .jp/youth/whitepaper/r01honpen/pdf_index.html.

Carr, David. 1986. *Time, Narrative and History.* Indiana University Press.

Conrad, Peter, and Joseph W. Schneider. 1992. *Deviance and Medicalization: From Badness to Sickness, Expanded ed.* Philadelphia: Temple University Press.

Council on Youth Affairs. 1989. "Sōgōtekina Seishōnen Taisaku no Jitsugen wo mezahite" [Toward the Realization of Comprehensive Youth Policy]. Accessed February 23, 2022. https://www.niye.go.jp/youth/book/files/items/1538/File/ sougouteki.pdf.

———. 1991. "Seishōnen no Mukiryoku, Hikikomori tō no Mondai Kōdō eno Kihonteki na Taiō Hōsaku" [Basic Measures to Deal with Youth Apathy, Hikikomori, and Other Problematic Behaviors: Toward the Development of Youth with Vitality]. Accessed February 16, 2022. https://www.ipss.go.jp/publication/j/ shiryou/no.13/data/shiryou/syakaifukushi/430.pdf.

Council for Youth Independence and Challenge Strategy. 2003. *Wakamono Jiritu Chōsen Puran* [*Plan for Youth Independence and Challenges*]. Accessed February 16, 2022. https://www5.cao.go.jp/keizai-shimon/minutes/2003/0612/ item3-2.pdf.

Dworkin, Ronald M. 1994. *Life's Dominion: An Argument about Abortion, Euthanasia, and Individual Freedom.* New York: Vintage Books.

Epston David, Michael White and Kevin Murray. 1992. "A Proposal for Re-Authoring Therapy: Rose's Revisioning of her Life and a Commentay." In *Therapy as Social Construction*, edited by S. McNamee, and K.J. Gergen. London: Sage Publications Ltd.

Erikson, Erik H. 1968. *Identity: Youth and Crisis.* New York: W. W. Norton & Company, Inc.

Esping-Andersen, Gøsta. 1990. *The Three Worlds of Welfare Capitalism.* Polity Press.

———. 1999. *Social Foundations of Postindustrial Economies.* Oxford University Press.

———. 2001. *Fukushi Kokka no Kanōsei: Kaikaku no Senryaku to Rironteki Kiso* [*Possibilities for the Welfare State: Strategies for Renovation and Their Theoretical Base*] edited and translated by Masao Watanabe and Keiko Watanabe. Sakurai Shoten.

Foucault, Michel. 1976. *La volonté de savoir (Histoire de la sexualité, Volume 1)* [*The will to Knowledge (The History of Sexuality, Volume 1)*]. Gallimard.

Frank, Arthur W. 1995. *The Wounded Storyteller: Body, Illness, and Ethics.* The University of Chicago Press.

Fukaya, Matsuo. 1985. "Miseijuku-shi Fuyōhō no Kiso teki Kōsatsu" [Basic Consideration of the Support Law for Immature Children]. *Kanazawa Hōgaku* 27, nos. 1 and 2: 199–236.

Furlong, Andy. 2008. "The Japanese Hikikomori Phenomenon: Acute Social Withdrawal among Young People." *The Sociological Review* 56, no. 2: 309–325.

Futagami, Noki. [2005] 2009. *Kibō no NEET* [*NEETs of Hope*]. Shinchō-sha.

Genda, Yūji. 2005. "NEET to Hikikomori" [NEET and Hikikomori]. *Kokoro no Kagaku* [*Science of Mind*] 123: 44–49.

Giddens, Anthony. 1984. *The Constitution of Society: Outline of the Theory of Structuration.* Polity Press.

———. 1991. *Modernity and Self-Identity: Self and Society in the Late Modern Age.* Polity Press.

Goffman, Erving. [1956] 1967. "The Nature of Deference and Demeanor." In *Interaction Ritual: Essays on Face-to-Face Behavior.* New York: Doubleday Anchor.

———. [1957] 1967. "Alienation from Interaction." In *Interaction Ritual: Essays on Face-to-Face Behavior.* New York: Doubleday Anchor.

———. 1967. *Interaction Ritual: Essays on Face-to-Face Behavior.* New York: Doubleday Anchor.

———. 1971. *Relations in Public: Microstudies of the Public Order.* New York: Basic Books.

———. 1974. *Frame Analysis: An Essay on the Organization of Experience.* Boston: Northeastern University Press.

Goodman, Roger. 1998. "The 'Japanese-Style Welfare State' and the Delivery of Personal Social Services." In *The East Asian Welfare Model: Welfare Orientalism and the State*, edited by Roger Goodman, Huck-Ju Kwon, and Gordon White. London: Routledge: 139–158.

Gotō, Michio. 2004. "Nihon-gata Shakai-hoshō no Kozō: Sono Keisei to Tenkan" [The Structure of Japanese-style Social Security: Its Fomation and Transformation]. In *Kōdo-Keizai-Seichō to Kigyō-Shakai* [*High Economic Growth and Corporate-Centered-Society*], edited by Osamu Watanabe. Yoshikawa-kōbun-kan.

———. 2012. "'Hitsuyō' Hantei Haijo no Kiken: Beisikku Inkamu ni tsuite no Memo" [The Danger of Excluding 'Needs' Judgments: A Note on Basic Income]. In *Besikku Inkamu ha Kyūkyoku no Shakaihosyō ka* [*Is Basic Income the Ultimate Social Security?*], edited by Toshihito Kayano. Horinouchi-Shuppan.

Hacking, Ian. 1996. "The Looping Effects of Human Kinds." In *Causal Cognition: A Multi-disciplinary Debate*, edited by D. Sperber, D. Premack, and A. J. Premack. Oxford University Press: 351–383.

———. 2002. *Historical Ontology.* Harvard University Press.

Hagiwara, Yasuhiro. 2001. "Waga Hikikomori-Taiken wo koete" [Beyond My Hikikomori Experience]. In *Gendai no Esupuri* [*Contemporary Esprit: Hikikomori*], edited by Seiei Mutō and Takeshi Watanabe, no. 403: 203–207.

Hamaguchi, Keiichirō. 2009. *Atarashii Rōdō Shakai: Koyō Sisutemu no Saikōchiku e* [*New Labour Society: Reconstructing the Employment System*]. Iwanami Shoten.

———. 2013a. *Wakamono to Rōdō: "Nyusha" no Shikumi kara Tokihogusu* [*Youth and Labour: Disentangling the Mechanism of "Entering Company"*]. Chuō Kōron Shinsha.

———, ed. 2013b. *Fukushi to Rōdō, Koyō* [*Welfare, Labor, and Employment*]. Minerva Shobō.

Hashikawa, Kensuke. 2021. "Chiiki Kyōsei Shakai Seisaku ni taisuru hihanteki Kentō to Kongo no Kadai ni kansuru Yobiteki Kōsatsu" [A Critical Review of

Community-Inclusive Society and a Preliminary Discussion of Future Issues]. *Kinjō Gakuin Daigaku Ronshū Shakai Kagaku-hen* [*Treatises and Studies by the Faculty of Kinjō Gakuin University, Studies in Social Sciences*] 17, no. 2: 31–40.

Hashimoto, Shin'ya. 2013. "Kingendai-Sekai ni okeru Kokka, Shakai, Kyōiku: 'Fukushi-Kokka to Kyōiku' toiu Kanten kara" [State, Society, and Education in the Modern and Contemporary World: From the Perspective of 'Welfare State and Education']. In *Fukushi-Kokka to Kyōiku: Hikaku-Kyōiku-shakaishi no Aratana Tenkai ni mukete* [*Welfare State and Education: Toward a New Development of Comparative Educational History*], edited by Teruyuki, Hirota, Shin'ya, Hashimoto, and Makoto, Iwashita. Shōwa-do.

Hayano, Toshiaki. 2015. "Daigaku-Zaiseki-chū no Miseinen-shi ni taisuru Oya no Fuyō-Gimu" [Parental Obligation to Support Adult Children in University]. *Hakuō Hōgaku* [*Hakuoh Review of Law and Politics*] 21, no. 2: 295–318.

Hayashi, Naomi. 2003. *Hikikomori nante Shitakunakatta* [*I Didn't Want to Be a Hikikomori*]. Sōshisha.

Headquarters for the Promotion of Support for the Development of Children and Youth. 2010. "Kodomo Wakamono Bijon" [Vision for Children and Youth]. Accessed February 23, 2022. https://www8.cao.go.jp/youth/suisin/pdf/vision .pdf.

———. 2016. "Kodomo Wakamono Ikusei Shien Suishin Taikō" [Policy Outline for the Promotion of Support for Children and Youth Development] Accessed February 23, 2022. https://www8.cao.go.jp/youth/suisin/pdf/taikou.pdf.

Headquarters for the Promotion of Youth Development. 2003. "Seishōnen Ikusei Shisaku Taikō" [National Youth Development Policy Outline]. Accessed February 16, 2022. https://www8.cao.go.jp/youth/suisin/yhonbu/taikou.pdf.

———. 2008. "Seishōnen Ikusei Shisaku Taikō" [National Youth Development Policy Outline]. Accessed February 16, 2022. https://www8.cao.go.jp/youth/suisin /taikou_201212/pdf/taikou_z.pdf.

Higuchi, Norio. 1988. *Oyako to Hō: Nichi-bei Hikaku no Kokoromi* [*Parents-Children and the Law: An Attempt at a Comparison of Japan and the United States*]. Kobun-do.

Higuchi, Akihiko. 2008. "'Hikikomori' to Shakaiteki Haijo" ['Hikikomori' and Social Exclusion]. In *"Hikikomori" heno Shakaigaku-teki Apurōchi: Media, Tōjisha, Shien-katsudō* [*Sociological Approaches to "Hikikomori": Media, Hikikomori Subjects, and Support Activities*]. Minerva Shobō.

Hikikomori UX Kaigi. 2019. "Kawasaki Sasshō Jiken nit suite (Seimeibun)" [About Kawasaki Murder Case (a statement)] Accessed February 23, 2022. http://blog .livedoor.jp/uxkaigi/190531_HikikomoriUxKaigi.pdf.

Hirata, Atsushi. 2020. "Minpō 877 Jō (Fuyō Gimusha) no Keifu to Kaishaku" [The pedigree and the interpretation of Civil Code Article 877]. *Meiji Daigaku Hōka Daigakuin Ronshū* [*Meiji Law School review*] 23: 1–39.

Hirayama, Yōsuke. 2011. *Toshi no Jōken: Sumai, Jinsei, Shakai-jizoku* [*The Condition of the City: Housing, Life, and Social Sustainability*]. NTT Publishing.

Hironaka, Masayoshi. 2003. "'Hikikomori' no Imi" [The Meaning of 'Hikikomori']. In *Hikikomoru Seishōnen no Kokoro: Hattatsu-rinsHō-shinrigaku-teki Kōsatsu*

[*The Mind of Withdrawn Youth: A Developmental Clinical Psychological Study*], edited by Yūko Okamoto and Kazuhiro Miyashita. Kitaōji Shobō.

Hirota, Teruyuki. 2013. "Fukushi-Kokka to Kyōiku no Kankei wo Dō Kangaeru ka" [How to Think about the Relationship between Welfare State and Education]. In *Fukushi-Kokka to Kyōiku: Hikaku-Kyōiku-shakaishi no Aratana Tenkai ni mukete* [*Welfare State and Education: Toward a New Development of Comparative Educational History*], edited by Teruyuki, Hirota, Shin'ya, Hashimoto, and Makoto, Iwashita. Shōwa-do.

Honda, Yuki. 2006. "'Genjitsu: 'NEET'ron toiu Kimyō-na Gen'ei" ['Reality': A Strange Illusion of 'NEET' Theory]. In *"NEET" tte Iuna! [Don't call us "NEET"!]*, edited byYuki Honda, Asao Naitō, and Kazutomo Gotō. Kōbunsha.

Honma, Yoshito. 2009. *Kyojū no Hinkon [Housing Poverty]*. Iwanami Shoten.

Horiguch, Sachiko. 2012. "Hikikomori: How Private Isolation Caught the Public Eye." In *A Sociology of Japanese Youth: From Returnees to NEETs*, edited by Roger Goodman, Yuki Imoto, and Tuukka Toivonen. Routledge: 122–138.

Inamura, Hiroshi. 1993. *Futokō, Hikikikomori Q&A [School Non-Attendance and Hikikomori Q&A]*. Seishin Shobō.

Inui, Akio, Akihiko Higuchi, Masahiko Sano, Maki Hiratsuka, Takeshi Hori, Yoshie Miura, and Andy Biggart. 2021. "Wakamono no Otona eno Ikō to Shakai Hoshō: Shūgyō to Rika, Kazoku Keisei wo meguru Nichi-ei Hikaku" [Youth Transition to Adulthood and Social Security: A Japanese-English Comparison of Employment, Leaving Home, and Family Formation]. *Shakai Seisaku Gakkai-shi [Social Policy and Labor Studies]* 13, no. 1: 120–31.

Ishikawa, Akane. 2013. "Seinen-ki ni okeru Kako no Trae-kata no Kōzō: Kako no Torae-kata-Shakudo no Sakusei to Datō-sei no Kentō" [The Structure of Perceiving the Past in Adolescence: Creation and Validity of the Past Perception Scale]. *Seinen Shingaku Kenkyu [Journal of Adolescent Psychology]* 24, no. 2: 165–181.

———. 2014. "Seinenki ni okeru Kako no Toraekata Taipu kara mita Mokuhyō Ishiki no Tokushō: Jikanteki Tenbō ni okeru Kako, Genzai, Mirai no Kanren" [The Relationship between the Past, Present, and Future in the Time Perspectives of Adolscents]. *Hattatsu Shinrigaku Kenkyū [The Japanese Journal of Developmental Psychology]* 25, no. 2: 142–150.

Ishikawa, Ryōko. 2006. "'Hikikomori' to 'NEET' no Kondō to sono Mondai: 'Hikikomori' Tōjisha heno Intabyū kara no Shisa" [Confusion of the Concepts of 'Hikikomori' and 'NEETs': Seen from the Perspective of People Who Regard Themselves as 'Hikikomori']. *Kyōiku Shakaigaku Kenkyū [The Journal of Educational Sociology]* 79: 25–44.

———. 2007. *Hikikomori no Gōru: "Shuro" demo "Taijin-kankei" demo naku [Goal of Hikikomori: Neither "Employment" nor "Personal Relation"]*. Seikyūsha.

Itō, Jun'ichirō, and Research Group on Community Mental Health Activities for Hikikomori. 2004. *Chiiki Hoken ni okeru Hikikomori eno Taiō Gaidorain [Guideline for Coping with Hikikomori in Community Health]*. Jihō.

JILPT (Japan Institute for Labour Policy and Training). 2011. *Rōdō Seisaku Kenkyū Hōkokusho No. 129: "Wakamono Tōgōgata Shakaiteki Kigyō" no Kanōsei to*

Kadai [*Labour Policy Research Report No. 129: Possibilities and Challenges of "Youth-Integrated Social Enterprises"*].

Kagawa, Mei, Hideyasu Kodama, and Shin'ichi Aizawa. 2014. "*Kōsotsu Tōzen Shakai" no Sengo-shi: Daredemo Gakkō ni Kayoeru Shakai ha Iji Dekiru no ka* [*Postwar History of 'Society Where High School Graduation is the Norm': Can a Society Where Everyone Can Go to High School Be Maintained?*]. Shin'yōsha.

Kamimura, Yasuhiro. 2015. *Fukushi no Ajia: Kokusai-Hikaku kara Seisaku-Kōsō e* [*Welfare in Asia: From International Comparisons to Policy Concepts*]. Nagoya Daigaku Shuppankai.

Kaneko, Sachiko. 2006. "Japan's 'Socially Withdrawn Youths' and Time Constraints in Japanese Society: Management and Conceptualization of Time in a Support Group for 'Hikikomori.'" *Time & Society* 15, no. 2: 233–249.

Kanō, Rikihachirō, and Naoji Kondō. 2000. *Seinen no Hikikomori: Shinri-Shakai-teki Haikei, Bōyri, Chiryō-enjo* [*Adolescent Hikikomori: Psychosocial Background, Pathology, and Treatment Support*]. Iwasaki Gakujutsu Shuppan.

Kariya, Takehiko. 1995. *Taishū Kyōiku Shakai no Yukue: Gakurekishugi to Byōdō Shinwa no Sengo-shi* [*The Future of Mass Education Society: The Postwar History of Gakureki-ism and the Myth of Equality*]. Chūō Kōron Sha.

Kasahara, Yomishi. 1988. *Taikyaku-Shinkei-shō: Mukiryoku, Mukanshin, Mukairaku no Kokufuku* [*Retreat Neurosis: Overcoming Apathy, Indifference, and Idleness*]. Kōdansha.

Katada, Kaori. 2017. "Tai-Hinkon Seisaku no Shin-Jiyūshugiteki Saihensei: Saiseisan Ryōiki ni okeru 'Jirtsu Shien' no Shosō" [Neoliberal Reforms of Anti-Poverty Schemes in Japan : Implications of "Self-Reliance Support" in the Reproductive Field]. *Keizai Shakai to Jendā* [*Journal of Feminist Economics Japan*] 2: 19–30.

Katsube, Reiko. 2016. *Hitori Bocchi wo Tsukuranai: Komyunitī Sōshal Wākā no Shigoto* [*No One Left Behind: The Work of Community Social Workers*]. Zenkoku Shakai Fukushi Kyōgikai.

Katsumata, Sachiko. 2008. "Kokusai Hikaku kara mita Nihon no Shōgaisha Seisaku no Ichiduke: Kokusai Hikaku Kenkyū to Hiyō Tōkei kara no Kōsatsu" [Japanese Policies for Persons with Disabilities in International Perspective: A Comparison using Expenditure Statistics]. *Kikan Shakai Hoshō Kenkyū* [*The Quarterly of Social Security Research*] 44, no. 2: 138–149.

Katsuyama, Minoru. 2001. *Hikikomori Karendā* [*Hikikomori Calendar*]. Bunshun-Nesuko.

———. 2011. *Anshin Hikikomori Raifu* [*A Safe Hikikomori Life*]. Ōta Shuppan.

Kawakita, Minoru. 2003. "'Hikokomori' no Enjo-ron to Ryōshin no Ichi: Kainyū no Konkyo to Sekinin wo megutte [Theory of Support and Parents' Position on 'Hikokomori': On the Basis of Intervention and Responsibility]." *Nagoya-daigaku Shakaigaku-ronshū* [*The Sociological Review of Nagoya University*] 24: 179–196.

———. 2004. "Hikikomori Oya no Kai no Soshiki Senryaku: 'Oya ga kawaru' toiu Kaiketsusaku no Sentaku" [Self-Help Groups of Parents with 'Hikikomori' Children and the Strategy of Self-Change]. *Gendai no Shakai Byōri* [*Journal of Social Problems*] no. 19: 77–92.

————. 2005. "Stōri toshite no Hikikomori-keiken" [The Hikikomori Experience as a Story]. *Aichi-kyōiku-daigaku Kyōiku-issen-Sōgō-Sentā Kiyō* [*Bulletin of the Center for Educational Practice, Aichi University of Education*] no. 8: 261–268.

————. 2006. "Kazoku-kai e no Sanka to Hikikomori no Kaizen: Minkan-shien-kikan ni okeru Shitsumon-shi Chōsa kara" [Participation in Family Associations and the Improvement of Hikikomori: From Questionnaire Surveys in Private Support Organizations]. *Aichi-kyōiku-daigaku Kyōiku-issen-Sōgō-Sentā Kiyō* [*Bulletin of the Center for Educational Practice, Aichi University of Education*] no. 9: 227–236.

————. 2008. "'Hikikomori' to Kazoku no Keiken" ['Hikikomori' and the Experience of Family]. In Ogino, Tatsushi, Minoru Kawakita, Kōji Kudō, and Ryūtaro Takayama, eds. 2008. *"Hikikomori" eno Shakaigakuteki Apurōchi: Media, Tōjisha, Shien Katsudō* [*Sociological Approaches to "Hikikomori": Media, Subjects, and Support Activities*]. Minerva Shobō.

KHJ. 2009. *"Hikikomori" no Jittai ni kansuru Chōsa Hōkokusho 6: NPO Hōjin Zenkoku "Hikkomori" KHJ Oya no Kai (Kazoku Rengōkai) ni okeru Jittai: "Hikikomori Chiiki Shien Sentā (Kashō)" ni nozomu Shien* [*Research Report on the Actual Condition of Hikikomori 6: Actual Condition in the NPO Zenkoku Hikomori KHJ Parents' Association: Support Needs for the 'Hikikomori Community Support Center (tentative name)'*]. Accessed February 16, 2022. https://www.khj-h.com/wp/wp-content/uploads/2018/05/08houkokusho.pdf.

————. 2010. *"Hikikomori" no Jittai ni kansuru Chōsa Hōkokusho 7: NPO Hōjin Zenkoku Hikikomori KHJ Oya no Kai ni okeru Jittai* [*Research Report on the Actual Condition of "Hikikomori" 7: Actual Condition in the NPO Zenkoku Hikikomori KHJ Parents' Association*]. Accessed February 16, 2022. https://www.khj-h.com/wp/wp-content/uploads/2018/05/tyousa_7.pdf.

————. 2016. *Hikikomori no Jittai ni kansuru Ankēto Chōsa Hōkokusho* [*Report of the Questionnaire Survey on the Actual Condition of Hikikomori*]. Accessed February 16, 2022. https://www.khj-h.com/wp/wp-content/uploads/2018/05/15houkokusho.pdf.

Kimoto, Kimiko. 2004. "Kazoku to Kigyō Shakai: Rekishi-teki Hendō Katei" [Family and Corporate Society: Historical Change Process]. In *Henbō suru Kigyō Shakai* [*Changing Corporate Society*] edited by Osamu Watanabe. Shunpō-sha.

Kimura, Tadafumi. 2015. "E. Goffuman no Hito-Yakuwari Zushiki Ron" [Erving Goffman's Argument about the Person-Role Formula]. *Shakaigaku Kenkyū* [*Sociological Research*] no. 95: 49–74.

Kitao, Tomohiko. 1986. "Ochikobore, Mukiryoku, Hikikomori [Drop-outs, Apathy, and Hikikomori]." *Kyōiku to Igaku* [*Education and Medicine*] 34, no. 5: 439–443.

Kobayashi, Shigeo. 1989. "Kodomo no Kakawari-Shōgai" [Involvement Disorders in Children]. In *Kodomo no Kakawari-Shōgai* [*Involvement Disorders in Children*], edited by Shigeo Kobayashi. Dōhōsha-shuppan: 2–27.

————. 1989. *Kodomo no Kakawari-Shōgai* [*Involvement Disorders in Children*]. Dōhōsha Shuppan.

Kojima, Taeko. 2016. *Q&A: Oyako no Hō to Jitsumu* [*Q&A: Law and Practice for Parents and Children*]. Nihon Kajo Shuppan.

Kondō, Naoji. 1997. "Hi-Bunretsubyō-sei Hikikomori no Genzai" [The Presence of Non-schizophrenic Hikikomori]. *Rinshō-seishin-igaku* [*Clinical Psychiatry*] 26, no. 6: 1159–1167.

———, ed. 2001. *Hikikomori Kēsu no Kazoku Enjo: Sōdan, Chiryō, Yobō* [*Family Support for Hikikomori Cases: Consultation, Treatment and Prevention*]. Kongō Shuppan.

Kondō, Naoji, Yoshikazu Kiyota, Yūji Kitabata, Yasukazu Kuroda, Mie Kurosawa, Motohiro Sakai, Homurasaki Fujinomiya, Natsuki Inomata, Hisae Miyazawa, and Ryōji Miyata. 2010. "Shishunki Hikikomori ni okeru Seishin Igakuteki Shōgai no Jittai Hāku ni kansuru Kenkyū" [Research on the Actual Condition of Psychiatric Disorders in Adolescent Hikikomori]. In *Kōsei Rōdō Kagaku-kenkyū-hi Hojokin Kokoro no Kenkō Kagaku-kenkyū Jigyō, "Shishunki Hikikomori wo Motarasu Seishinka-shikkan no Jittai Hāku toSeishin-igaku-teki Chiryō, Enjo Sisutemu no Kōchiku ni kansuru Kenkyū (Shunin Kenkyūsha, Saitō Kazuhiko)": Heisei-21-nendo Sōkatsu Buntan Kenkyū Hōkokusho* [*MHLW Grants-in-Aid for Scientific Research on Mental Health, "Research on the Actual Condition of Psychiatric Disorders Causing Adolescent Hikikomori and the Construction of Psychiatric Treatment and Support Systems (Principal Investigator: Kazuhiko Saitō)" FY 2009 Summury Report of Researches*]: 67–102.

Kosugi, Reiko. 2004. "Jakunen-mugyōsha no Jittai to Haikei: Gakkō kara Shokugyō Seikatsu e no Ikō no Airo toshiteno Mugyō no Kentō" [The Reality and Background of the Increase in the Number of Jobless Youth: An Examination of Joblessness as a Standstill of the Transition from School to Occupational Life]. *Nihon Rōdō Kenkyū Zasshi* [*The monthly journal of the Japan Institute of Labour*] 533: 4–16.

Kudo, Kōji. 2008. "Yure-ugoku 'Hikikomori'" [Changing Hikikomori]. In Ogino, Tatsushi, Minoru Kawakita, Kōji Kudō, and Ryūtaro Takayama, eds. 2008. *"Hikikomori" eno Shakaigakuteki Apurōchi: Media, Tōjisha, Shien Katsudō* [*Sociological Approaches to "Hikikomori": Media, Subjects, and Support Activities*]. Minerva Shobō.

———. 2013. "'Hikikomori' Shakai Mondai-ka ni okeru Seishin Igaku: Bōryoku, Hanzai to 'Risuku Suiron'" [Psychiatry and a Social Problem of 'Hikikomori': Violence, Crime, and 'Risk Reasoning']. In *Hōhō toshite no Kōchiku-shugi* [*Constructionism as a Method*], edited by Nobutoshi Nakagawa and Manabu Akagawa. Keisō Shobō.

Kudō, Sadatsugu. 1997. *Ōi, Hikikomori: Sorosoro Soto e Dete Miyōze* [*Hey, Hikikomori: It's Time to Go Outside*]. Potto Shuppan.

Kuramoto, Nobuhiko. 2002. "Hikikomori to Jiko-ai: Mō-hitotsu no Aidentiti" [Hikikomori and Narcissism: Another identity]. *Rinshō Shinrigaku* [*Journal of Clinical Psychology*] 2, no. 6: 763–768.

Malagón-Amor, Á., D. Córcoles-Martínez, M. M. Martín-López, and P. Pérez-Solà. 2015. "Hikikomori in Spain: A Descriptive Study." *International Journal of Social Psychiatry* 61, no. 5: 475–483.

Maruyama, Yasuhiko. 2014. *Futōkō Hikikomori ga Owaru Toki: Taikensha ga Tōjisha to Kazoku ni kataru Rikai to Taiō no Michishirube* [*When School Non-Attendance and Hikikomori End: A Guide for Understanding and Coping, as Told by a Peson Who Has Experienced Them for People in Those Situations and Their Families*]. Raifu Sapōto Sha.

MHLW. 2003. *Jūdai, Nijūdai wo chūshin to shita "Hikikomori" wo meguru Chiiki Hoken Katsudō no Gaidorain: Seishin Hoken Fukushi Sentā, Hokenjo, Shichōson de donoyōni Taiō suru ka* [*Guideline for Community Mental Health Activities Regarding Hikikomori, Focusing on People in their Teens and Twenties*]. Accessed March 4, 2022. https://www.mhlw.go.jp/topics/2003/07/tp0728-1.html.

———. 2010. *Hikikomori no Hyōka Shien ni kansuru Gaidorain* [*Guideline for the Evaluation and Support of Hikikomori*]. Accessed Feburary 10, 2022. https://www.mhlw.go.jp/file/06-Seisakujouhou-12000000-Shakaiengokyoku-Shakai/0000147789.pdf.

———. 2015. "Seikatsu-konkyū-sha Jiritsu Shien Seido Shōkai Rīfuretto" [Leaflet Introducing the System for Supporting the Independence of Those in Need]. Accessed August 16, 2016. https://www.mhlw.go.jp/stf/seisakunitsuite/bunya/0000073432.html.

———. 2018. "Seikatsu Konkyūsha Jiritsu Shien Seido to Kankei Seidotō tono Renkei ni tsuite" [Cooperation between the System for Supporting the Independence of Those in Need and Related Systems]. March 16, 2022. https://www.mhlw.go.jp/content/000362597.pdf.

———. 2019a. "Hikikomori Jōtai ni aru kata ya sono Gokazoku eno Shien ni mukete" [Toward a Support for People in Hikikomori Condition and Their Families]. February 23, 2022. https://www.mhlw.go.jp/content/12000000/000522281.png.

———. 2019b. "Hikikomori Shien Shisaku no Hōkōsei to Chiiki Kyōsei Shakai no Jitsugen ni mukete (Shichōson Seminā Shiryō)" [Direction of Policies to Support Hikikomori and Realization of a Community Inclusive Society (Material for Municipal Seminar)]. Accessed February 14, 2022. https://www.mhlw.go.jp/content/12600000/000554777.pdf.

———. 2022a. "Seikatsu Konkyūsha Jiritsu Shien Seido: Keii" [The System for Supporting the Independence of Those in Need: Its details]. Accessed February 23, 2022. https://www.mhlw.go.jp/stf/seisakunitsuite/bunya/0000057342.html.

———. 2022b. "Seikatsu Konkyūsha Shien Seido: Seido no Shōkai" [The System for Supporting the Independence of Those in Need: Introduction of the System]. Accessed on February 23, 2022. https://www.mhlw.go.jp/stf/seisakunitsuite/bunya/0000073432.html.

Ministry of Land, Infrastructure, Transport and Tourism. 2013. *Kokudo Kōtsū Hakusho 2013: Wakamono no Kurashi to Kokudo Kotsū Gyōsei* [*White Paper on Land, Infrastructure, Transport and Tourism 2013: Young People's Lives and Land, Infrastructure, Transport and Tourism Administration*]. Nikkei Insatsu.

Miyake, Atsuko. 1999. "Oya no Miseijukushi in taisuru Fuyō Gimu ni tsuite" [On the Obligation of Parents to Support Their Immature Children]. *Hōsei Kenkyū* [*Journal of Law and Politics*] 66, no. 2: 733–759.

Miyamoto, Michiko. 2015a. "Jakunen Mugyōsha to Chiiki Wakamono Sapōto Stēshon Jigyō" [NEETs and Local Youth Support Stations]. *Kikan Shakai Hoshō Kenkyū* [*The Quarterly of Social Security Research*] 51, no. 1: 16–26.

———. 2015b. "Ikōki no Wakamonotachi no Ima" [Youth in Transition]. In *Subete no Wakamono ga Ikirareru Mirai wo: Kazoku, Kyoiku, Shigoto kara no Haijo ni Kōshite* [*Toward a Future where All Youth Can Live: Against Exclusion from Family, Education, and Work*], edited by Michiko Miyamoto. Iwanami Shoten.

Miyamoto, Tarō. 2013. "Seikatsu Hoshō no Atarashii Senryaku" [New Strategy for Life Security]. In *Seikatsu Hoshō no Senryaku: Kyōiku, Koyō, Shakai wo Tsunagu* [*Strategy for Life Security: Connecting Education, Employment, and Society*], edited by Tarō Miyamoto. Iwanami Shoten.

———. 2017. "'Chiiki Kyōsei Shakai' ron to Kyōsei Hoshō no Senryaku" [Theory of 'Community Inclusive Society' and Strategy for Ensuring Inclusion]. *Niji: Kyōdō Kumiai Keiei Kenkyūshi* 660: 7–16.

Momose, Yū. 2010. *Shōgai Nenkin no Seido Sekkei* [*System Design of the Disability Pension*]. Kōseikan.

Moriguchi, Hideshi, Naho Naura, and Kazumasa Kawaguchi, eds. 2002. *Hikikomori Shien Gaido* [*A Guide to Supporting Hikikomori*]. Shōbunsha.

Mukaiyachi, Ikuyoshi, and Urakawa Beteru no Ie. 2006. *Anshin shite Zetsubō dekiru Jinsei* [*Life with No Worries to Despair*]. NHK Shuppan.

Nagatomi, Natsue, and Hideshi Moriguchi. 2005. *Shutoken-ban Syakaiteki Hikikomori Gaido Mappu* [*Guide Map for Supporting Social Withdrawal in the Tokyo Metropolitan Area*]. Yui Puranningu.

Nakamura, Karen. 2013. *A Disability of the Soul: An Ethnography of Schizophrenia and Mental Illness in Contemporary Japan*. Cornell University Press.

NHK Kurōzu Appu Gendai. 2011. Episode 2997, "Hataraku no ga Kowai: Aratana Hikikomori [Fear to Work: New Hikikomori]." Aired Febrary 3, 2011, on NHK.

Nichter, Marck. 2018. "Idioms of Distress." In *The International Encyclopedia of Anthropology*, edited by Hilary Callan. John Wiley & Sons, Ltd.

Niko Niko Pedia. 2022. "Hikikomori." Last modified January 28, 2022. https://dic .nicovideo.jp/a/%E5%BC%95%E3%81%8D%E3%81%93%E3%82%82%E3%82 %8A.

Nishimura, Yukimitsu. 2014. "Henbō suru Wakamono no Jiritsu no Jittai" [Changing Realities of Youth Independence]. *Kikan Shakai-hoshō Kenkyū* [*The Quarterly of Social Security Research*] 49, no. 4: 385–396.

Nomura, Masami. 2014. *Gakurekishugi to Rōdō Shakai: Kōdo Keizai Seichō to Jieigyō no Suitai ga motarashita mono* [*Meritocracy and Employee Society: Effects of High Economic Growth and the Decline of Self-Employment*]. Minerva Shobō.

Ochiai, Emiko. 2013. "Kea Daiamondo to Fukushi Rejimu: Higashi Ajia, Tōnan Ajia Roku Shakai no Hikaku Kenkyū" [Care Diamond and Welfare Regimes: Comparative Study of East and Southeast Asian Six Societies]. In *Shinmitsuken to Kōkyōken no Saihensei: Ajia Kindai kara no Toi* [*Reorganization of Intimate and Public Spheres: Questions from Asian Modernity*], edited by Emiko Ochiai. Kyōto Daigaku Gakujutsu Shppankai.

OECD. 2015. *Education at a Glance 2015: OECD Indicators*. OECD Publishing.

———. 2016. *Economic Policy Reforms 2016: Going for Growth Interim Report*. OECD Publishing.

———. 2022. "Social Expenditure." Accessed January 26, 2022. https://stats.oecd .org/Index.aspx?QueryId=33415.

Ogino, Tatsushi. 2008a. "'Hikikomori' to Taijin Kankei: Tomodachi o meguru Konnan to sono Igi" ['Hikikomori' and Interpersonal Relations: Difficulties over Friends and Their Meaning]. In Ogino et al. 2008.

———. 2008b. "'Hikikomori' to Seishin Iryō: Minkan Shien Katsudō no Shisa suru mono" ['Hikikomori' and Psychiatory: Implications of Private Support Activities]. In Ogino et al. 2008.

Ogino, Tatsushi, Minoru Kawakita, Kōji Kudō, and Ryūtaro Takayama, eds. 2008. *"Hikikomori" eno Shakaigakuteki Apurōchi: Media, Tōjisha, Shien Katsudō [Sociological Approaches to "Hikikomori": Media, Subjects, and Support Activities]*. Minerva Shobō.

Okuda, Yūichiro. 2008. "Daigakusei no Jikanteki Tenbō no Kōzō ni kansuru Kenkyū: Kako, Genzai, Mirai no Manzokudo no Sōtaiteki Kankei ni Chakumoku shite" [A Study of Time Perspective Structure in University Students: Approach from Relations of Past, Present and Future]. *Maebashi Kyoai Gakuen Daigaku Ronshū [Kyōai Gakuen University Journal]* 8: 13–22.

———. 2013. "Daigakusei no Jikanteki Tenbō no Jidaiteki Hensen: Wakamono wa Mirai wo Egakenaku nattano ka" [A Historical Transition of the Undergraduate's Time Perspective: Can the Undergraduates Picture the Future in the Postmodern?]. *Maebashi Kyoai Gakuen Daigaku Ronshū [Kyōai Gakuen University Journal]* 13: 1–12.

Ōsawa, Mari. 2007. *Gendai Nihon no Seikatsu Hoshō Sisutemu: Zahyō to Yukue [Life Security System in Contemporary Japan: Coordinates and Future]*. Iwanami Shoten.

———. 2013. *Seikatsu Hoshō no Gabanansu: Jendā to Okane no Nagare de Yomitoku [Governance of Life Security: Deciphering Gender and Money Flows]*. Yuhikaku.

Ovejero, Santiago, Irene Caro-Cañizares, Victoria de León-Martínez, and Enrique Baca-Garcia. 2014. "Prolonged Social Withdrawal Disorder: A Hikikomori Case in Spain." *International Journal of Social Psychiatry* 60, no. 6: 562–565.

Polanyi, Karl. 1944. *The Great Transformation*. Farrar and Rinehart.

Saitō, Takuya, Shizuko Kameyama Barnes, and Yoshiko Nishimatsu. 2003. "Amerika ni okeru Futōkō eno Apurōchi: Futōkō to Kaifuku wo Enjo suru Hōteki na Wakugumi" [Approaches to School Non-Attendance in the United States: A Legal Framework for Supporting School Non-Attendance and Recovery]. *Seishinka Chiryōgaku [Journal of Psychiatric Treatment]* 18, no. 12: 1433–1440.

Saitō, Tamaki. [1998] 2013. *Hikikomori: Adolescence without End*. Translated by Jeffrey Angles. University of Minnesota Press.

———. 2002. *"Hikikkomori" Kyūshutsu Manyuaru [Resucue Manual for "Hikikomori"]*. PHP Kenkyūjo.

———. [2003] 2016. *Hikikomori Bunka-ron [Cutural Theory of Hikikomori]*. Chikuma Shobō.

———. 2012. "Hikikomori Mondai no Shakaigakuteki Sokumen to Shien no Arikata ni tsuite" [The Sociological Aspects of the Hikikomori Problem and How to Support It]. In *Hikikomori ni deatta ra: Kokoro no Iryō to Shien [When You Meet a Hikikomori: Psychosomatic Treatment and Support]*, edited by Kazuhiko Saitō. Chūgai Igaku-sha.

———. 2015. "'Hikikomori' wo meguru Saikin no Dōkō" [Recent Trends Surrounding 'Hikikomori']. *Rinshō Seishin Igaku [Clinical Psychiatry]* 44, no. 12: 1565–1571.

Sakurai, Toshiyuki. 2003. "Hikikomori Keikensha no Katari ni kansuru Ichi Kōsatsu: Erikuson no "Aidentiti" Gainen wo Tegakari ni" [A Study on Talk by Individuals Who Have Experienced Social Withdrawal]. *Ōsaka Daigaku Kyōikugaku Nenpō* [*Osaka University Annals of Educational Studies*] 8: 223–234.

Satō, Yōsaku. 2005. "Wakamono Jiritsujuku no Genba kara: Satō Yōsaku san ni kiku" [From the Field of Youth Independence School: Interview with Yōsaku Satō]. *Zen'ei* [*Vanguard*] 736: 143–151.

Sawada, Yuki. 2021. "'Hikikomori' Tōjisha no Jiko Teiji to Aidentiti wo meguru Mondai" [Self-presentation and Identity of 'Hikikomori' People]. *KG Shakaigaku Hihyō* [*KG Sociological Review*] 10: 1–13.

Schutz, Alfred. [1953] 1962. "Common-sense and Scientific Interpretation of Human Action." In *Collected Papers I: The Problem of Social Reality*, edited by Maurice Natanson. Martinus Nijhoff.

———. [1957] 1964. "Equality and the Meaning Structure of Social World." In *Collected Papers II: Studies in Social Theory*, edited by Arvid Brodersen. Martinus Nijhoff.

Schutz, Alfred and Thomas Luckmann. 1973. *The Structures of the Life-World, Volume 1*, translated by Richard M. Zaner and H. Tristram Engelhardt Jr. Northwestern University Press.

Sekimizu, Teppei. 2016. *"Hikikomori" Keiken no Shakaigaku* [*Sociology of the Hikikomori Experience*]. Sayūsha.

———. 2021. "'Hikikomori' and Dependency on Family: Focusing on Father–Son Relationships." *International Journal of Japanese Sociology* 30, no. 1: 182–196.

Shimizu, Masayuki. 2003. "Hikikomori wo Kangaeru" [Thinking about Hikikomori]. *Seishin Igaku* [*Clinical Psychiatry*] 45, no. 3: 230–234.

Shiokura, Yutaka. [1999] 2002. *Hikokomoru Wakamono-tachi*. Asahi Shinbun Shuppan.

———. [2000] 2003. *Hikokomori*. Asahi Shinbun Shuppan.

———. 2002. "'Hikikomori' wo miru Shiten" [A Viewpoint on 'Hikokomori']. *KōKō Seikatsu Shidō* [*High School Educational Guidance*] 152: 6–13.

Social Security Council. 2013. *Seikatsu Konkyūsha Shien no Arikata ni kansuru Tokubetsu Bukai Hōkokusho* [*Report of Special Subcommittee on Livelihood Support for Those in Need*]. Accessed February 16, 2022. https://www.mhlw.go.jp/stf/shingi/2r9852000002tpzu-att/2r9852000002tq1b.pdf.

Socio-Economic Productivity Center. 2007. *NEET no Jōtai ni aru Jakunensha no Jittai oyobi Shiensaku ni kansuru Chōsa Hōkokusho* [*Report on the Actual Conditions and Support Measures for Youth in NEET Status*]. Accessed February 16, 2022. https://www.mhlw.go.jp/houdou/2007/06/dl/h0628-1b.pdf.

Sugiyama, Masahiko. 1989. "Shakaiteki Hikikomori" [Social withdrawal]. In Kobayashi 1989.

Suzuki, Tomoyuki. 2002. "Yakusha Atogaki [Translator's Postscript]." In *Kidutsuita Monogatari no Katarite: Shintai, Yamai, Rinri* [*The Wounded Storyteller: Body, Illness, and Ethics*]. Yumiru Shuppan.

Tachibanaki, Toshiaki. 2005. *Kigyō Fukushi no Shūen: Kakusa no Jidai ni Dō Taiō subeki ka* [*The End of Corporate Welfare: How We Should Respond to the Era of Disparity*]. Chūō Kōron Shinsha.

Tajan, Nicolas. 2021. *Mental Health and Social Withdrawal in Contemporary Japan: Beyond the Hikikomori Spectrum.* Routledge.

Takaoka, Ken. 2001. "Aru Hikigeki: Inamura Hiroshi to Saitō Tamaki" [A Tragicomedy: Hiroshi Inamura and Tamaki Saitō]. *Seishin Iryō, Dai 4 ji* [*Psychiatry, Forth*] 24, no. 99: 72–80.

Takayama, Ryūtarō. 2008. "Futōkō kara 'Hikikomori' e" [From School Non-Attendance to 'Hikikomori']. In Ogino et al. 2008.

Takegawa, Shōgo. 2007. *Rentai to Shōnin: Gurōbaru ka no naka no Fukushi Kokka* [*Solidarity and Recognition: Welfare State in Globalization and Individualization*]. Tokyo Daigaku Shuppankai.

Takikawa, Kazuhiko. 2012. *Gakkō ni Iku Imi, Yasumu Imi: Futōkō tte Nandarō?* [*The meaning of Going to School and Being Absent from School: What is School Non-Attendance?*]. Nihon Tosho Sentā.

Tanabe, Yutaka, ed. 2000. *Watashi ga Hikikomotta Riyū* [*The Reason I Withdrew*]. Bukkuman Sha.

Tanaka, Chihoko. 1996. *Hikikomori: "Taiwa suru Kankei" wo Torimodosu tame ni* [*Hikikomori: To Restore "Dialogic Relationships"*]. Saiensu Sha.

———. 2001. *Hikikomori no Kazoku Kankei* [*Family Relations of Hikikomori*]. Kōdansha.

Toivonen, Tuukka. 2012. "NEETs: The Strategy within the Category." In *A Sociology of Japanese Youth: From Returnees to NEETs*, edited by Roger Goodman, Yuki Imoto, and Tuukka Toivonen. Routledge: 139–158.

Tomita, Fujiya. 1992. *Hikikomori kara no Tabidachi: Tōkō Shūshoku Kyohi kara "Ningen Kyohi" suru Kodomotachi tono Kokoro no Kiroku* [*Departure from Hikikomori: A Heartfelt Record of Children Who Refuse to Go to School, Refuse to Work, and Reject Human Beings*]. Hāto Shuppan.

———. 1994a. *Yomigaetta Kazoku no Kizuna: Tōkō Shūshoku Kyohi suru Kodomotachi* [*Revived Family Ties: Children Who Refuse to Go to School or Work*]. Hāto Shuppan.

———. 1994b. *Hikikomori to Tōkō Shūshoku Kyohi Q&A* [*Hikikomori, School and Job Refusal Q&A*]. Hāto Shuppan.

———. 1995a. *Kodomo-tachi no Angō: Tōkō Shūshoku Kyohi suru Kodomotachi* [*Children's Codes: Children Who Refuse to Go to School or Work*]. Hāto Shuppan.

———. 1995b. *Shikiri Naoshi no Junrei: Tōkō Shūshoku Kyohi* [*Pilgrimage to a Fresh Start: School and Job Refusal*]. Hakujusha.

Tokyo Metropolitan Youth and Public Safety Headquarters. 2009. *Hikokoruru Wakamono-tachi to Kazoku no Nayami: Heisei 20-nendo Jakunensha Jiritsu Shien Chōsa Kenkyū Hōkokusho* [*Youth and Family Concerns: FY 2008 Survey Report on Independence Support for Youth*]. Tokyo Metropolitan Government.

Tsutsui, Miki, Junri Sakurai, and Yuki Honda, eds. 2014. *Shūrō Shien wo Toinaosu: Jichitai to Chiiki no Torikumi* [*Reconsidering Job Support: Local Governments and Communities Initiatives*]. Keisō Shobō.

Uchida, Hiroaki. 2005. "A Study of the Necessity for the School Social Work Who Sees from Operating Analysis of Child Guidance Office." *Nagano Daigaku Kiyō* [*Bulletin of Nagano University*] 26, no. 4: 1–17.

Ueyama, Kazuki. 2001. *"Hikikomori" datta Boku kara* [*From Me, Who Was a "Hikikomori"*]. Kōdansha.

———. 2002. "Kojin deha naku: Hikikomori Tōjisha no Koe" [Not as Individual: A Voice of a Hikikomori Subject]. *KōKō Seikatsu Shidō* [*High School Educational Guidance*] 152: 28–33.

———. 2006. "Iyō ni Jiyū / traumatic freedom." Freezing Point. Posted January 17, 2006. Accessed Febuary 14, 2022. http://d.hatena.ne.jp/ueyamakzk/20060117/p2.

Ushijima, Sadanobu, and Jōji Satō. 1997. "Hi-Bunretsubyō no Hikikomori no Seishin Rikidō" [Psychodynamics of Nonschizophrenic Hikikomori]. *Rinshō Seishin Igaku* [*Clinical Psychiatry*] 26, no. 9: 1151–1156.

Uzuhashi, Takafumi. 2011. *Fukushi Seisaku no Kokusai Dōkō to Nihon no Sentaku: Posuto "Mittsu no Sekai" Ron* [*International Trends of Social Welfare Plicy and Japanese Choice: Theory of the Post-Three-Worlds*]. Hōritsu Bunka Sha.

Watanabe, Osamu. 2004. "Kaihatsu Shugi, Kigyo Shakai no Kōzō to sono Saihensei" [Developmentalism, Structure of Corporate Society and its Reorganization]. In *Henbō suru Kigyō Shakai* [*Changing Corporate Society*], edited by Osamu Watanabe. Shunpō-sha.

Yamamoto, Kiyoko. 2009. "Kazoku Kihan no Henka to Shakai Seisaku: Rōjin to Kodomo no Shakaiteki Ichi wo megutte" [Changes in Family Norms and Social Policy: The Social Position of the Elderly and Children]. *Sonoda Gakuen Joshi Daigaku Ronbunshū* [*Sonoda Gakuen Women's University Journal*] 43: 27–40.

Yamamoto, Kōhei. 2013. *Tomo ni Iki Tomoni Sodatsu Hikikomori Shien: Kyōdōteki Kankeisei to Sōsharu Wāku* [*Hikikomori Support Where We Live Together, We Grow Up Together: Cooperative Relationship and Social Work*]. Kamogawa Shuppan.

Yamazaki, Mitsuhiro. 2019. "'Wagakoto Marugoto' Chiiki Kyōsei Shakai no Honshitsu to Kadai" [The Essence and Challenges of 'Taking It Personally, Entirely' Community Inclusive Society']. *Shakai Hoshō* [*Social Security*] 472: 9–15.

Yoshikawa, Hiroshi. 2012. *Kōdo Seichō. Nihon wo kaeta 6000 nichi* [*High Economic Growth: Six Thousand Days that Changed Japan*]. Chūō Kōron Shinsha.

Yoshikawa, Takehiko. 2010. "Seishin Igaku kara mita 'Hikikomori': Naikakufu ga jisshi sita Honchōsa to Koremade no waga Kuni ni okeru 'Hikikomori' Chōsa no Sai ni furete" ['Hikikomori' from the Perspective of Psychiatry: In Reference to the Differences between this Survey Conducted by the Cabinet Office and Previous 'Hikikomori' Surveys in Japan]. In *Wakamono no Ishiki ni kansuru Chōsa (Hikikomori ni kansuru Jittai Chōsa) (Gaiyō-ban)* [*Survey on Youth's Consciousness (Fact-finding Survey on Hikikomori) (Summary Version)*], edited by Cabinet Office. Accessed February 17, 2022. https://www8.cao.go.jp/youth/kenkyu/hikikomori/pdf/gaiyo.pdf.

Youth Affairs Headquarters. 1990. *Heisei Gannen-ban Seishōnen Hakusho: Seishōnen Mondai no Genjō to Taisaku* [*White Paper on Youth: Current Situation and Measures for Youth Problems*]. Ōkurashō Insastu-kyoku.

Index

Page references for figures and tables are italicized.

163

About the Author

Teppei Sekimizu is associate professor of sociology in the Faculty of Social Welfare at Rissho University, Japan. He is the author of *Sociology of Hikikomori Experience* (2016) and coauthor of *Sociology of Hikikomori and Their Family* (2018) and the *Hikikomori White Paper* (2021) in Japanese. He has also published more than 10 articles about the hikikomori issue including "'Hikikomori' and dependency on family: Focusing on the father-son relationship," *International Journal of Japanese Sociology* (2021), and "The foundations of support relationship for Hikikomori people: Self-determination, shared-determination, and self-definition," *Schutzian Research*, vol. 9 (2017).

www.ingramcontent.com/pod-product-compliance
Lightning Source LLC
Chambersburg PA
CBHW022318280326
41932CB00010B/1149